Love Your Skin

Expert Skin Care Secrets Exposed

Cover Art by Marcus Bieth of Mark3GraphicDesigns.com
Edited by Justin H. Phillips

Manufactured in the United States of America

Love Your Skin

Expert Skin Care Secrets Exposed

By Nicci Leigh L.E.

DEDICATION

This book is dedicated to all of my clients throughout the years who have allowed me to learn about the skin by working with theirs. Without you, this book would not exist. To anyone who struggles with their skin on a daily basis, may we all face the world together, with skin we love to live in…

-Nicci Leigh

TABLE OF CONTENTS

Love Your Skin

Preface:

Feel the Love

You deserve to love your skin. You should be able to look at your face in the mirror and be pleased with what you see. You should wake up every morning and watch the hands of time moving backward instead of forward, and see a radiant glow in your skin. If you cannot currently say you "Love Your Skin" in this way, you will be able to after you finish this book and begin implementing the "Love Lessons" into your daily skin care regimen. It is possible to have skin you love, you just have to know the right things to do for it.

I have a unique and deep understanding of the skin and a prolific career working one on one with clients in multiple areas of the skin care industry. I am honored to say, as a professional skin care therapist, my personal perspective on how to treat the skin has helped thousands of women transform theirs. I have written this book to share the way I see the skin so that you, too, can learn how to transform yours.

It's your face. It's the only one you've got and you can have perfect skin, no matter what. Yes, I said perfect. No matter what age or current condition your skin in. Yes, you can turn back the clock with the right knowledge. You can have clear skin. No, you do not have to suffer from skin you are unhappy with.

I will share what I've learned throughout my career in the beauty industry, and what I teach my aesthetic students who have gone on to have careers as top skin care professionals. You will learn what the pros know in this easy-to-understand guide. This is not a brief discussion of skin care like you may find in a magazine article or on a website. It is a complete in-depth guide for all ages and skin types.

That being said, skin care alone could be considered a 'dry' topic. I can't say that every woman is knocking down the romance books or classic novels on her bookshelf to get to the one on 'how to care for your skin.' I thought using the concept of 'loving your skin' would resonate better, since this typically isn't something that the majority of women can say they do. When a client walks through the door of my practice, generally there are two things I take from our consultation:

They do not currently love their skin.

They do not have a full understanding of how to properly care for it.

I didn't either before becoming an aesthetician, and I was already (as you know) a product junkie! Because I suffered from acne and other concerns since puberty, I know what it's like to not love your skin!

I use a 'no nonsense,' 'straight talk' approach to information. It is not intended to lessen the value of the information, but rather to cut through the fluff. I have found there is a large number of women who find skin care, and the multitudes of products and treatments available, difficult to understand. These are the women who are looking for a way to make sense of the massive subject of skin care, who want that radiant glow that gets you compliments like, " Wow, you really have gorgeous skin!" or "No, you can't be _____ years old! You look so young!" Be prepared to hear these if you don't currently.

I've used "Love and Relationships" as a theme for this book. I drew this parallel because love and relationships are things most women can relate to and have experience with. These experiences can easily be associated with the relationship you have with your skin. I use comparisons like this to make the topic fun and memorable so the information doesn't just go in one ear and out the other. Trust me, you won't forget about free radicals when I'm done with them!

This is not a book that is going to tell you, "You don't have to do x,y,z, to get great skin. You only have to do this one easy thing." Because that would be a lie. Skin care is no different from anything else: if you want results, you've got to put the work in. It's not one simple thing you will do that will give you skin you love. It's a combination of small things. Committing to doing these things, over time, is the secret...

It's similar to working out. There isn't one easy, effortless thing you can do, and have a perfect body (okay, for a few, there may be). For the rest of us, we know we have to work at it, and we either do or we don't. Unfortunately, the older we get, the more work we have to put into our face and our bodies.

I am not just going to tell you what to do—there are plenty of magazine and web articles to do that. I want to help you understand why you need to do it. I believe it is like the saying, "Knowledge is power." If you understand how and why to care for your skin, you will not only like doing it, you will love to.

Skin care is a multi-billion dollar a year industry. I see a trend or demand for products and treatments that will "do it all." Quick, easy, effortless…that's what we want. Why is this? Don't women deserve to take the time to care for their face and body? Are we supposed to be so busy that we need one product or treatment to take care of everything? In many countries outside of the United States, skin care is an accepted and celebrated part of their culture and plenty of time is devoted to it. Many European women receive weekly facials, and view it as maintenance rather than a luxury. You deserve to take the time to care for your skin, too. My hope is that by helping you understand it like a professional, you will feel empowered to do so.

I am hell-bent on getting you to love your skin. I want the information offered to sink in and stay with you long after you've read it, so I've layered the information within each chapter, building one on top of the next. Please read this guidebook from beginning to end, rather than skipping around. This will give you the best opportunity to make the most of it for you, personally. Get ready to fall in love with your skin!

Love Lesson 1

A Healthy Skin Relationship

In the same way that dental health isn't purely cosmetic, neither is skin care. Yet many people still view it as such. Nor is beauty only skin deep. For those who are unhappy with their skin, it goes deeper than just the surface, affecting their self-confidence. When you love yourself, it shows on the outside. When you love your skin, you feel it on the inside.

Your perspective of your skin, what it is, and its importance, is the first step in developing a healthy relationship with it. When you think of your skin as a living organ, which it is, it changes what you believe it's capable of, and how you care for it.

What do we know about the skin? The skin is the largest living organ of our body. It's made up of layers of dead cells, live cells, collagen and elastin fibers, nerves, pigment, and glands, to name just a few components. All of these things can be damaged and malfunction (just like a relationship!). All of these things can be repaired or improved (unlike some relationships!). You only get one skin. You live in

1

it from the day you are born until you the day you die. It's the only one you've got so you should know how to care for it and ultimately love it.

To have a healthy relationship with your skin, you must understand what makes it tick. This basic knowledge will get the relationship started. From the surface of your skin, down to the muscles beneath it, it contains:

The Epidermis: five layers of skin cells—the top two or three of which, depending on the area of the body, are dead. The bottom layer is living, and the in between layer is like a "Zombie" layer: half dead, half living. These layers combined are only as thick as a sheet of paper!

Under that is the Dermis (live layer) made up of: nerves, sweat glands, oil glands, hair follicles, blood vessels, pigment (color) cells, collagen (plumping) fibers, and elastin (stretchy) fibers.

Under these things is the sub-layer: adipose (fat) cells, and then your muscles attached to the bone.

All of these things, when damaged or not functioning properly, are the source of skin's problems. All of these things, when functioning properly, are the source of healthy, radiant skin. Everything that shows up on the surface of your skin has a direct connection with something in the aforementioned paragraph: skin, pigment, collagen, elastin, and fat cells; oil and sweat glands; and hair follicles. Our goal is to get all your skin's components as healthy as they can be. Get in the habit of thinking of your skin on a cellular level, not just as one entity as a whole. Think about how each thing you do will affect your skin cells individually. This perspective will drastically change your relationship with it.

Love Lesson # 2

Free Radical Love

Triangle

Know who your enemy is. This may be the most important lesson in skin care and relationships. "A good defense is the best offense." Heard that one, before? If you know who and what to look out for, you can save yourself the pain of a broken heart, or in our case a damaged cell. I'm leading with this lesson, to get right to the core of what causes the majority of skin problems: the enemy. I read a book years ago called What Smart Women Know by Steven Carter and Julia Sokol. It helped me to understand what I had learned the hard way: I was wasting my time in relationships with men who were bad for me. Once I could identify them, I could avoid them and spend my time identifying the ones who were right. I found one about a year later, and we are now happily married! Sometimes, just a change of perspective can make all the difference.

In this skin care lesson, we will discuss how to identify enemies of your skin, stay away from them, and protect your cell relationship, or "single" cells if you are not currently in a commitment!

I am sure you've heard the term "free radicals." It is commonly used in the health and nutrition world, and often by vitamin supplement companies. You may also have an idea that they are not good for you, but you don't know why, or what significance they have regarding your skin. I am also quite sure you are familiar with the infamous love triangle story of Angelina, Brad, and Jennifer. Let me preface this whole bit by saying: I am a HUGE Angelina fan, I think she is a goddess (and has great skin, too!), but I am a fan of the other two, as well. So, there is NO personal preference applied when using this analogy. It just made perfect sense and came off-the-cuff, in a night class when my students seemed to be nodding off during the free radical lesson. It was just too good to pass up...

Free radicals are created within your body by numerous sources, the most common offenders being the sun, stress, toxins like cigarette smoke, pollutants in the air and foods we eat, pesticides, preservatives, artificial colors and additives, byproducts of chemicals in plastics, and cleaners. Basically anything synthetic or unnatural, or highly aggressive (like the sun), produces free radicals. Even your body's own biological functions and inflammation produce them. The love triangle unfolds from there...

Free radicals are what cause skin damage. They can damage any of the components within your skin. Your number one task is to protect your skin from them, and reverse the damage they have already done.

Here's where the Angelina / Brad / Jen love triangle comes in: a free radical is created from a highly energetic source capable of mutating cells (mentioned above). The free radical (Angelina—sorry, girl!), is a rebellious, powerful cell that is missing an electron (uneven #) and needs to find (steal or take) an electron from a normal, healthy cell which has an even amount of electrons (Brad & Jen). The healthy cell couple are just going about their everyday lives when along comes this wild, magnetic free radical (Angelina) cell. It so badly needs to replace the electron that it is missing that it breaks the bond in the healthy cell (Brad / Jen marriage) and steals an electron (Brad) for herself, leaving the formerly healthy cell (Jen) now broken hearted and damaged.

The free radical now has a new partner (Brad) and together they can go on and multiply, making free radical babies. The formerly healthy cell (Jen) is left alone, confused as to what the hell just happened.

Do you want this going on inside of your skin? Unfortunately, it's happening all the time. How, then, can it be prevented? With protection, both external and internal. Let's start with external first. This is comparable to what we are used to hearing termed "preventive." Stay away from anything capable of producing free radical Angelinas. Eliminate the opportunity for your cells to be close to them. I.e. Don't let your cell do a kick-ass spy movie with them! Translated this means: Stay out of the sun, don't smoke, don't drink, and eat clean. I know this is near impossible unless you are a nun or never plan to go on vacation again. Even nuns go on vacation. (I saw them on a beach in Mexico, myself!)

Do your best to stay away from any chemicals or synthetic products like Styrofoam, plastics, toxins, pollutants, et cetera. All the common sense stuff that we know is bad for us. You've heard this spiel before, so I will leave the rest of it up to someone else (I've listed some in the Resources section if you're interested). The truth is: Put your (Brad) cell in harm's way or near a free radical (Angelina) and be prepared to hear me say, "I told you so." Damage control will need to be done. How can the damaged cell repair its broken heart? Plenty of wine, yoga, and trips to Cabo? Kinda, sorta. We'll get to that later…

The second line of defense against the Angelina free radical is internal protection (close internal). Imagine if you had something you could place around or inside of the Brad and Jen cell that would make it invisible to the Angelina free radicals, if they just happened to be in each other's proximity. Would you do it? Of course you would!

The invisibility shield is "antioxidants," a term you are most likely also familiar with. You see, another term for an Angelina free radical is "Super-oxide." It's able to 'oxidate' (destroy, age, diminish) cells, and oxidation is the aging process. Any breakdown of cells equals aging. Any protection and repair of cells equals anti-aging. Aging means your cell (Brad) will end up sporting a funky goatee!

Here's a better example of oxidation everyone is familiar with: when you cut a piece of fruit and it sits out, exposed to open air (oxygen), it turns brown. You may also know that if you add lemon juice and/or sugar to a fruit salad it prevents the fruit from turning brown.

7

Back to the invisible antioxidant shields. When you introduce various antioxidants to your cells, you give your Brad cells the external and internal invisibility shields. Angelina can't even see them. She will tire out, and go away. If all the cells in your body are protected, the Angelinas will be powerless and disappear. You may be thinking: "What if I don't have any invisibility shields?" Well, then your precious fruit, or healthy cell relationship, is in jeopardy.

I'm anticipating your next thought to be, "Where can I get these invisibility shields?" You can get them from three main sources:

Externally from topical skin care products

Internally from dietary supplements

Internally from the foods you eat

Sounds easy enough, right? There is, however, a disclaimer: I am not a nutritionist or physician so please seek a professional in these areas before making any dietary changes. I am highly familiar with topical antioxidants, so I can advise you in this area, but as for antioxidants as supplements and food, I've included the Love Lesson "Feed Your Skin" later in the book, based on my education as a licensed skin care therapist, to get you started. I've also included additional reading and websites in the "Resources" section at the end of the book. More in-depth information can also be found at your local health food store.

ANTIOXIDANTS AND USAGE:

Vitamin C (L-Ascorbic Acid)

This is a BIG DOG in the realm of invisibility shields, likely the most effective one. It has muscle. Vitamin C comes in many forms: L-ascorbic acid, Citric acid, Bioflavinoids, Ester-C, and Ascorbic Palmitate being the most common ones. The only form capable of permeating the cell wall and getting inside of the Brad / Jen cell is L-ascorbic acid. It is also a more advanced, and sometimes more expensive, form of vitamin C, but it is worth it. Vitamin C is the common enzymatic cofactor in the production of collagen and a powerful reducer of the reactive oxides (free radicals). It fights and destroys them. In a cat fight with Angelina free radicals, L-ascorbic acid will win, hands down.

There are many topical L-ascorbic products on the market. I will recommend several brands later in the section on serums and anti-aging, I've also included a recipe you can make at home in the Love Lesson "DIY Skin Care."

How to use topical vitamin C: You only need to apply it (serum) in the morning, every other day. AM is the ideal time for vitamin C since this is when cells need protection. Think of it like this: Generally, your Brad cells are only exposed to Angelina free radicals during the day, and not at night while he is home, in bed. The L-ascorbic acid remains active in your skin for up to 24 hours, that's why you only need to apply it every other day. The exception to this rule is when you are on vacation, or outdoors for a prolonged period. Anytime the Brad cells will have their shirt off and a greater chance of exposure to Angelina free radicals, you will need your invisibility shields in full force.

Vitamin E

Another powerful antioxidant that acts as an invisibility shield is Vitamin E. It protects the cells from not only free radicals, but skin cancer, too. It's most effective in its natural alcohol form rather than its acetate form. It increases the effectiveness of sunscreens if applied to the skin at least 20 min before SPF application. You can buy vitamin E oil at your local health food store, or online. You can take vitamin E internally as well as vitamin C to support its use for skin treatment. Vitamin E boosts the effectiveness of vitamin C and regulates the next antioxidant we will be discussing, vitamin A, which can be very aggressive depending on which form it is in. Incorporate vitamin E into your protection and prevention plan and you will now have two guard dogs for your cells.

Vitamin A

Another BIG DOG is Vitamin A, also known as **Retinol** (in its most potent natural form), Adaptalene and Tretinoin. Vitamin A is in a league of its own. It is the Incredible Hulk of antioxidants because of its power, and it can often be too strong. It is the only substance in this realm that is able to not only penetrate the cell walls going directly into the cells, but it can travel through all tissues of the body including the blood stream. Because of this it has many more uses other than protection and invisibility. It is used to restructure and remove the top dead layer of cells right down to the live cell layer. When used as a protective antioxidant, vitamin A works best in small doses in serums or creams, and used in conjunction with C and E.

Additional antioxidants to include in your diet, supplements and skin care products:

Vitamin B, D3, K, F & H

Coenzyme Q10, Alpha Lipoid Acid (ALA)

Copper, Oligomeric Proanthocyanidin (pine bark), Grape Seed Extract

Green Tea, Resveratol, Beta Glucans & Polysaccharides (yeast), Amino Acids, Glutathione

With enough experience it is possible to look at a client's skin and have a good idea of what it is lacking internally and externally, and what it needs to regain its healthy state. When your skin is lacking the proper antioxidants, whether in your skin care regimen or diet, it will not have that healthy glow because it is utilizing its own resources and nutrients to protect itself from the free radicals. This diminishes the normal functions it needs, to have that glow on the inside and out. Getting back to our love triangle, if you provide the skin with invisibility shields it will be stronger

and have more time to focus on its own biological reproductive needs....enough said.

There are several other things to consider, besides antioxidants, that will ensure your cell relationship is not going
to stray. Here are a few more:

Water

When your cells are hydrated, they are resilient. If the
Brad cells would have been drinking plenty of water, they
would have been able to ward off Angelina's advances.
Drink half of your body's weight, in ounces, per day. In the
Love Lesson "Water, My Love" I will discuss the affects water has on our skin, and some delicious ways to get hydrated.

Oxygen

Increasing the oxygen uptake in the cells boosts the
skin's metabolism. Our skin has a metabolism like our
body's, regarding the breakdown of food into energy. We all
know that as we age, our metabolism slows. The same is
true for our cells and their ability to function when they are
trying to ward off harmful substances and toxins. Their
normal metabolism slows down. Increasing the oxygen in
the cells increases their metabolism.

You may be wondering why it's so important to increase the cells' metabolism. Anabolism is the term for the metabolic process that builds our cells—builds more cell tissue, to be exact. We want to build more healthy cells. We want to increase and support Brad and Jen's, well...when the cells absorb water, nutrients, and oxygen, they reproduce.

Back to oxygen; here's the easiest ways to increase your oxygen levels:

Breathe deeper! We spend most of our time in our mind, thinking and analyzing everything. When we are constantly in our mind, we are most likely holding our breath. Pay attention and see for yourself. When you are working, driving, at the store shopping, you are thinking about what happened yesterday, or what you have to do later that day, and you are not in the present, breathing—like you should be. Breathe more, breathe deeper, and your cells we receive more oxygen. Not just your skin cells, but all the cells in your body. Your complete metabolism will increase. A quick anatomy and physiology lesson: cells are singular, groups of cells make up tissues, groups of tissues make up organs, groups of organs make up body systems. Increasing the health and metabolism of the cells increases your overall health.

Exercise

Exercise to increase oxygen in your cells. Any type of exercise from walking to highly cardiovascular aerobic exercises will do. Even one minute of exercise every hour like jumping jacks, squats, push-ups or jogging in place will keep your metabolism up and oxygen flowing to the cells.

Yoga uses its own unique breath work system during the entire practice. It teaches you how to breathe deeper into your middle and lower abdomen, using your full lung capacity—instead of shallow breathing which only uses the top half of your lungs. Breathe deep into your abdomen and not just your upper chest area and a greater exchange of oxygen for carbon dioxide occurs. Yogic breathing can also help you incorporate deeper, conscious breathing into your everyday life and activities. Take a yoga class, or buy a DVD or book for home use. Do whatever you can do, even if it's minimal. Years ago, I was shopping for a yoga mat at a department store and a woman came up to me and said, "You have great skin, you must do yoga. Everyone who I know who does yoga is beautiful. I think I'm going to try it." She walked away before I could even respond. Any yoga is good yoga.

Yoga also regulates the endocrine system, which controls secretions in your body. These secretions affect metabolism, mood, sebum production, appetite, and sex drive, to name a few. When out of balance, these things can be either: hyperactive (too much), or hypoactive (too little). Yoga brings them back into normal, balanced function.

We've discussed things you can do to internally and externally protect your cells' healthy relationship. What if your cell already has a broken heart and has suffered previous damage at the hands of a free radical? What is Jen to do? Remember the wine, yoga, and trip to Cabo we mentioned earlier? That is exactly what she did, and you should, too! When a cell has been damaged by a destructive free radical, it's now missing an electron and is unbalanced. An unbalanced cell has the potential to spiral out of control and take other cells down with it. DON'T WAIT to heal a cell's broken heart. The longer you wait, the greater chance its unstable state will disrupt other cells. Instead, the wine (symbolic for antioxidants), yoga (strength, balance, and detoxification), and Cabo (relaxation and stress management), can help a cell rebound and heal itself. Yes, heal itself. When a cell has everything it needs, it can return itself to a natural state of homeostasis (balanced health). This is like what Jen did.

Remember this section when we discuss anti-aging; specifically, turning back the hands of time, in upcoming Love Lessons.

The truth is, we all have had our hearts (cells) broken. Everyone's skin has been damaged. All the measures mentioned to protect your cells from Angelina free radicals are the same things you do to heal a broken hearted cell if she does take away your Brad cell. Rest well knowing he will have plenty on his hands with their multiplying brood of cells, anyway. Your Jen cell can enjoy the healthy, single cell life!

I hope you don't mind me having a bit of fun with this Love Lesson. If the analogy has helped you to view your skin in a different way, then I am happy. The following "Love Lessons" will give you more tools to help you love your skin.

Love Lesson #3

Sun Worship

It is no secret that the sun is bad for our skin. We've all gotten that memo. What most women may not exactly know is why, so they still sneak a bit of sun worship in! "Sun exposure," just to clarify, does not only imply sun bathing or the use of a tanning bed. It refers to ANY time your skin is exposed to daylight. Sunny, cloudy, Canada, Brazil, or in between. All three hundred and sixty-five days of the year. It makes no difference, and here's why: UVA and UVB rays melt the delicate fibers and cells of your skin whenever they come in contact with it.

Have you ever had an elastic pair of underwear or bra that had been through the drier one too many times? If so, you will know that the stretchy material has lost its original shape. It is now loose and less pliant. Maybe you have had the same thing happen to a bathing suit or other fabric left outside in the sun for too long? They also lose their elasticity, and their color fades. Your skin is just like these fabrics, only more sensitive and delicate because it is a living material.

The collagen (plumping and thickening) and elastin (stretchy) fibers of your skin melt when exposed to the sun. Just like the bathing suit, bra, and panties, once they've lost their shape and elasticity they will never regain it. Let me repeat that last part: When your skin's collagen and elastin fibers are melted from sun damage they will never go back to their original state. This is what I consider when I don't feel like putting on SPF or another form of skin protection: melted face or no melted face?

Your Face vs. Your Butt

Here's another way to think about it: Most of the skin care schools use a text book by Milady's. I recall a section on sun exposure that had a photo of a bare bottomed baby (a typical old fashioned baby picture). There were also two other photos: One of the face and the other the backside, of that baby eighty years later as an elderly woman. What do you think had changed: her face, her backside, or both? As you can imagine her face had changed drastically. There were deep visible lines, wrinkles, loss of firmness, age spots, et cetera. In contrast, the tone and texture of the skin on her bottom did not show a significant difference. Not the overall shape of her behind, but the actual skin. The reason for this is that her face had 80+ years of exposure to the sun and elements. Her bottom, because it was covered by clothing, had little to none. Does this mean you have to cover your face? Yes, and no.

Let's look at the different types of the sun's rays—UVA and UVB—and what they have to do with your skin. UVA is the abbreviation given to the specific portion of the ultra violet rays responsible for most of the wicked mess we've mentioned in the bra and panty discussion. UVA stands for Ultra Violet Aging. I was floored when I first learned that. Aging? Yes, the same rays that give us our beautiful glowing tans, has the word "aging" right there, in its very name. These rays penetrate through ALL layers and components of the skin, muscle, right down to the bone! They are the ones that melt the tissue fibers, mutate cells, and produce Angelina free radicals.

The other ray, UVB, is short for Ultra Violet Burning. Yes, it's that simple, also. These rays have a shorter reach than UVA rays, and fry only the top layers of the skin, and cause a sunburn. You may be reading this chapter during a season where you aren't getting much sun exposure and feel the information isn't relevant to helping you get skin you love now. If so, consider this: one of the worst culprits of sun exposure year round happens in the car. It is a well known fact to skin therapists and dermatologists that most individuals' skin damage is greater on the left side of their face, from the exposure to UVA light through the driver's side window of the car! Brown spots, crow's feet, loss of firmness...very often, these are much worse on the left side of the face. All I can suggest, besides using an SPF every day, is to use your sun visor! I never allow the sun to beat down on the left side of my face while driving. It annoys my husband and children because I am constantly readjusting the visor (even when I am on the passenger side). I don't care if I look silly to everyone else with my big Audrey Hepburn shades on and sun visor down on an overcast day! It's worth lessening the risk of sun-induced cancer and skin damage, and keeps you looking younger, longer. Use it! Sun exposure also occurs indoors, if you sit next to a window at work, for example. Just running errands and going in and out of the car qualifies as sun exposure, too!

Another effect of the sun that concerns many women is uneven pigmentation. The presence of dark spots (hyper-pigmentation) and light spots (hypopigmentation) on the skin can be caused from sun damage. Here's another analogy to help you understand what's happening within, when you have sun spots on your skin. Think of a pigment cell (melanocyte) like a spider with its eight legs. When a healthy melanocyte produces color or pigment (melanin), it distributes it equally out the eight legs, which carry the color to the skin's surface and results in an even skin tone.

When the pigment spider cell is damaged, its legs become broken and the pigment can no longer travel through them. Because of this, all the pigment will be forced to use what legs may still be functioning, resulting in a concentrated dark spot on the skin's surface, or no pigment on the skin's surface if all the spider's legs are broken.

Like our previous recipe on how to heal a broken cell, you need to remove the destructive factors (sun), introduce repairing ones (antioxidants) and protect them from future damage (SPF), and your spider cells legs can heal and return to their normal, even pigment production!

It is my hope that this Love Your Skin tutorial on sun exposure helps you understand exactly what is going on when you are worshipping, and not worshipping, the sun. We have all heard the lip service paid to the benefits of the sun, like vitamin D production. I even saw an episode of the TV show "Wife Swap" where a woman gazed at the sun for food. So I will leave the list of benefits to someone else, and further try to shed some light (ah, the pun) on the subject so you can better prepare yourself for a future of ageless skin. Here's what I recommend:

If you are going to sun bathe, COVER YOUR FACE! Did you hear me scream that loud enough? The skin on your face, neck, and décolleté (chest), is more delicate than other parts of your body, and much more susceptible to damage than other areas which contain thicker cells and more collagen and elastin. So, when you are at the pool or on vacation, never mind who's watching and place a small hand towel, or even use your cover-up (worst-case-scenario), and lay it over your FACE and NECK! Who cares what those other sunbathers and vacationers think? They do not have to wear your face in twenty-five years, you do. You will have the face of a twenty-five year old when you are fifty, and they may not. It is your face, the only one you've got, so protect it! If you are past twenty-five or have already become friendly with UVA and UVB rays, it's never too late. We will discuss how to repair it in the Love Lesson on premature aging. For now, we'll continue with SPF coverage:

SPF Rules

You need to know which SPF is right for you. SPF is the abbreviation for Sun Protection Factor. If you were to go outdoors without sunscreen: Take the amount of time before your skin would burn (i.e. 30 min) and multiply that by the sunscreen number, say SPF 30. So, 30 minutes x 30 SPF = 900 minutes. 900 minutes ÷ 60 minutes in an hour = 15 hours of protection. Wow. That's if you could withstand 30 minutes in the sun without burning. Realistically, that would be an individual who has medium pigmented skin. A light skinned individual may burn after only 5-15 minutes in the sun, so a SPF 30 would give you 7.5 hours outdoors (maximum) before it no longer offered protection. Keeping in mind that SPFs lessen in effectiveness once applied to your skin, after you sweat or swim, I don't think the current system is always accurate. Over the last several years, the FDA has approved SPFs from Europe that maintain their integrity the entire time they are on your skin. They are also chemical based. I cover the differences in SPFs in the Love Lesson "Proper Protection."

If you cover your face like you cover your ass, you will have a face like a babe until the end!

Expert Tip

Skin care professionals often perform a Pinch Test to check the amount of elasticity in the skin. You can, too. Pinch any area of your skin and gently pull it outward, then release it. The quicker is snaps back, the more elastin fibers the skin has. The slower the skin returns to its natural shape, the less elastin the skin contains and, likely, the more damage that has been done to that area. Focus your efforts on repairing and protecting this skin if you are not, already.

Remember, it's never too late to return your skin to, or keep it in, a youthful state! Keep reading...

Love Lesson #4

Water, My Love

We have heard, "To have great skin you must drink plenty of water," for years. This is another lesson where women may not exactly understand why. Here is the truth about why your skin loves water:

More water equals less oil. This may not seem like a big deal unless you have oily, combination, or acneic skin, then, it's a huge deal. Your skin produces oil in an attempt to moisturize itself. It didn't get the memo that breakouts and shine are not helpful. Thanks, but no thanks, oil glands. Water tricks your oil glands into thinking your skin is "moisturized" already. If they believe your skin doesn't need oil, they won't produce it. When you are dehydrated, your skin cells are lacking the amount of water they need to function properly, so your oil glands kick in to help out. You can trick that pesky oil output by drinking at least half your body weight in ounces, per day. If you weigh 130 pounds, you would need to drink 65 ounces of water, which would equal around four average size bottles of water or six glasses of water, per day. That's not so bad, is it? If you only drink water when you are thirsty, you are not drinking enough. Drink it even when you are not thirsty.

Toxins

"I love what you do, but you know that you're toxic." Thanks, Britney Spears, for the truth. Everyday toxins enter your skin cells. What goes in needs to come back out. Without plenty of water, those harmful toxins have plenty of time to hang out with your precious skin cells. Flush them out! If you don't like the taste—or lack of taste—of water, there are plenty of flavor enhancers on the market like. Some are naturally flavored, but most are not. Use them sparingly, until you can go without. Look for ones that contain skin loving vitamins. Some of my favorites are "Karma Water"www.drinkkarma.com and
"Fix" www.yourdailyfix.com.

You are water, my love. Between one half and two-thirds of your body is made up of water. Your skin is the largest organ of the body. You connect the dots. Your skin needs water to function properly! Quite often, many skin concerns and conditions will disappear when you are regularly hydrated. Redness, Rosacea, skin sensitivity, dryness, fine lines, irritations, excessive oiliness, and breakouts are just a few on the list of issues that can be resolved when you start drinking enough water. Drink in the love! Here are a few delicious, spa-inspired water recipes:

FLAVORED SPA WATER RECIPES

Citrus Mint

Spring or Purified Water

Fresh Citrus Fruit Slices: Orange, Lemon, Lime or Combination

2-4 Fresh Mint Leaves

Pineapple Strawberry

Spring or Purified Water

Fresh Pineapple Slices

Strawberry Slices

Cucumber Slices

Berry Burst

Spring or Purified Water

Fresh Raspberries

Fresh Blueberries

Fresh Lemon Slices

2-4 Fresh Basil Leaves

Place fruits and/or herb leaves into a water pitcher. You can muddle the fruit and leaves if you wish your water to have more flavor. Pour water into pitcher and keep refrigerated. Serve with or without ice and garnish with fruit or fresh leaves.

These waters are filled with skin loving antioxidants and are several of my favorite recipes. Have fun and experiment to discover new ones of your own!

Love Lesson #5

Product

Comparisons

Have you tried products from every brand sold at the drugstore and department store? Do you have a bathroom shelf or drawer of unused products? Have you bought products from a local spa or gotten them from your dermatologist? How do you know if the $8.00 face cream is as good as the $80.00 one? Does it matter where you get them? How do the products you buy measure up, and why?

We've already discussed the health and functions of your skin. But before we jump into discussing skin care regimens to support those functions, let's take a moment to compare the differences in skin care products. The differences are mainly based on where you buy them from. This inside information of the cosmetic industry will empower you to make the best choices regarding what you put on your skin.

To my "soap and water" friends: many women refrain from using skin care products because they are unsure which products to use and when. Also, they really don't want to spend the money on it if it's not right for their skin, or isn't going to work. I can sympathize. I hope that these clarifications will empower you to make informed choices.

The FDA (U.S Food and Drug Administration) regulates the amount of certain active ingredients such as hydroxy acids, formulations, and retinols that a product contains, based on who sells them and where they are available for purchase. This is interesting and important because it's information most cosmetic consumers are unaware of, and it affects how much of a change the product can make in your skin.

A simple definition of an "active" ingredient would be: "Part of a substance, respective of the amount, that helps to achieve performance objectives and has a direct effect in restoring, correcting, or modifying biological functions." In other words, it gets the job done. Have you often wondered if the creams, potions, and lotions you are putting on your face are doing what they are supposed to? Whether they are or not is directly connected to how much of an active ingredient the manufacturer puts, and is allowed to put, into the cosmetic.

Love Note: The terms "Active" and "Inactive," when referring to ingredients, is typically reserved for the drug industry only, but are commonly used in the beauty industry for simplicity's sake. They do not actually affect function, but rather the appearance and health of our skin. The terms "Functional" and "Performance" are the appropriate terms used when identifying cosmetic ingredients, but will be substituted with "active" and "inactive," subsequently.

Here's how product categories measure up in order of lowest active amount to highest: (This information may be disputed as, active levels vary from State to State and are based upon each one's specified laws and regulations. The FDA regulations are limited. This information is based off my professional experience working with and for cosmetic companies in all the following categories and is intended for educational purposes only.)

Drugstore / Retail

This includes any product you are able to walk into a store and buy off the shelf. Product companies like Neutrogena, Oil of Olay, and Cetaphil. These companies are only allowed to manufacture and sell products that contain 4-10% "active" ingredients, which means 96-90% are inactive ingredients like fillers and binders such as water, waxes, and preservatives. Why is this? Because if anyone can buy it, anyone can use it. What if someone bought a product that was too powerful, or it wasn't appropriate for their skin type? It could result in an adverse reaction or negative side effect. It can be compared to the availability of "over the counter" drugs versus "prescription" drugs, with regard to their strength and potential effects.

The problem is that most women need products that will do more for than their skin conditions than these products can. They buy retail products expecting to see drastic results that the companies may lead women to believe they will receive, but the products just aren't capable of enacting.

The Plus: Drugstore products are lower in price. These companies are industry giants with enormous resources and advertising campaigns. They have come a long way in an attempt to compete with "Cosmeceuticals" (products that claim to combine cosmetic and pharmaceutical benefits; such as anti-aging products) on the market. Also, the retailers who sell them often have return policies that allow you to take the product back if you are unhappy with it.

The Problem: Many women buy drugstore brands because they are familiar with the manufacturer's name. Quite often they are unsure whether it is the right product for their skin, or even making a difference, since they have no one to consult with. Because of the lesser amount of active ingredients, many women are "wasting" precious opportunities each day to be using something that does make the desired changes in their skin. Women are unaware that there are products available that, if they spent just a few dollars more and found the right fit for their skin, could be getting far more results than they've come to expect.

Department Store

This category would constitute any product company that you would need to buy from a sales representative at a cosmetic counter, like: Clinique, Chanel, and Estee Lauder.

Brands where you have an opportunity to consult with a trained representative for that company. Here there is a higher degree of probability that the consumer will find a better match for their skin type. Because of this, the level of active ingredients is raised to 7-10%, leaving the other 90-93% as the inactive ingredients like binders and fillers.

The Plus: You can discuss your skin's concerns with a consultant from that company, who will likely be able to help you to select the correct products for your skin. Products can be applied to your skin for demonstration purposes so you can feel and test them before you buy them. These companies are also working hard to compete with the "cosmeceutical" companies and drugstore brands, so their research and formulas continue to advance.

The Problem: Department store products are usually significantly higher in price due to the commission they pay to the sale representatives, and the cut given to the retail stores where they are sold. Often these companies do not offer a return or exchange program, so if you get the product home and are unhappy with it, you are stuck with it. The last problem I have with the department store companies is rarely discussed: in an attempt to protect their product formulas, they rename their ingredients with names they have patented. These names are exclusive to their company and professionals and consumers have no idea what this ingredient really is. Often, the ingredients they rename are synthetic variations of natural ingredients or slight variations of active ingredients used by other companies. These mystery ingredients, in my opinion, can be very deceptive.

Professional Grade

This category includes products that can only be obtained from a licensed skin care professional such as an aesthetician, registered nurse, dermatologist, or plastic surgeon. You would be familiar with these product lines if you have had a facial at a spa, or a treatment at a medical spa, or dermatologist's office. Brands like Murad, Perricone, SkinCeuticals, and Dermalogica. Products from these companies are not prescription medications, however, professional grade companies do offer the "cosmeceuticals" we have previously mentioned.

Professional grade products require the person recommending them to have an advanced knowledge of the skin's functions and also to have earned a degree or license. For this reason, the level of certain active ingredients can range between 30-70% varying by the State they are sold or applied in. Therefore, much less of the product consists of inactive ingredients.

These products do facilitate greater reactive tendencies and visible differences in the skin. Because of this, they cannot be sold without the assistance of a skin care professional, since the wrong match for your skin could cause unwanted changes or reactions. For example, a professional grade acne product, if used on sensitive skin, could cause excessive redness, dryness, or burning to the skin. The higher the level of "active" ingredients, the more the product can do for you.

The Plus: If you want to see a significant change in your skin, professional grade products and the recommendation by a professional will increase the likelihood that you will find the correct product matches that will make a difference for your skin. Having a professional who knows your skin is beneficial when you have any questions about the products you are using. Because of their higher ingredient concentrations, you can use a smaller amount and they will last longer than lesser concentrated products.

The Problem: Professional grade products are not as readily available as drugstore and department store brands. Consumers are less familiar with professional products because they are required to be sold in a Spa or office setting only. People do not generally walk into a spa or doctor's office and buy a product off the shelf (you legally can't) without undergoing a treatment or consultation from a qualified skin care professional.

Several beauty retail chains like Sephora and Ulta now carry some of the larger professional grade product lines. (It's similar to grocery stores carrying the professional brands of hair products that used to only be available at a hair salon.) These beauty retailers hire an aesthetician for consultation, and this allows them to offer the higher grade skin care.

Professional lines usually carry a slightly to significantly higher price tag than drugstore brands, due to the higher level of active ingredients, and the use of a "middleman." Skin care companies sell to a wholesaler, who sells to the spa, who sells it to you. However, the prices are typically in line with department store brands, so they are affordable to everyone.

Prescription Grade

The only products in this category are ones that can be classified as "medicinal," meaning it contains a drug or substance used to treat or prevent a condition or disease: topical products used by, or only obtained from, a physician or nurse practitioner. Because of this, they contain upwards of 70% concentration of active ingredients and / or medicine. These products are capable of creating immediate, if not permanent, changes to the skin, its functions and structure. Prescription acne creams, topical retinols, antibiotics, hydroxy acids, and products containing these substances are included in this category. Some of the drug companies manufacture skin care lines only available from a physician, like Retin-A, Renova®, Latisse®, and Vaniqa®, just to name a few.

The Plus: If you have a serious condition of the skin, these products may be necessary, and the only thing to remedy the problem. Cystic acne, infections, rosacea, dermatitis, vitiligo, pigmented, excessive hair growth, adhesions, injuries, and significant aging are all common concerns treated by these types of products.

The Problem: Often, consumers seek out these products from a physician when another grade of skin care product would be sufficient for their skin. Some consumers believe that dermatologists' products and recommendations are the be-all end-all, and will only use what their dermatologist recommends. This isn't always the best perspective. Your doctor may recommend you lose weight or exercise more, but your doctor isn't going to be your personal trainer. It's the same with skin care. The symptom is often a result of a concern that can be remedied by improving the health of your skin.

To summarize this Love Lesson, the more interaction you have with a licensed professional when you buy your products, and the more education they have, the more "active" the product will be, and the more chances it has to make changes in your skin.

This information is not meant to persuade or dissuade you in any way as to what type of products you choose, but rather to help you better understand what's on the market so you can make an informed, educated decision about what you put on your face. I have a saying when it comes to skin care products, "If it works, it works. If it doesn't work, it doesn't." Meaning: you should see a difference in your skin whether you are using an $8.00 product or an $80.00 one. If it is the right product for you, you will see a difference. If you don't see changes—stop using it. There is NO such thing a specific period of time that you should give a product before you see results. This is hype. If the product is going to work, it will work right away, and it will keep working, with the results continuing to show as time goes by. Also, if a product once worked and it stops working—S-TOP USING IT. Your skin needs change and it no longer meets your skin's needs. It's time to move on to a new skin relationship!

Love Lesson #6

Product Ingredients

Before we get to the Love Lessons regarding how to care for your skin, let's learn how to evaluate your product's ingredients. I've always been a label reader. Call me a cosmetic geek, but I have been fascinated by exactly what is inside of those bottles and jars, and the potential they may or may not have to give me the results I am looking for. As a skin therapist, and educator to future aestheticians, I need to have a deep understanding of product ingredients and the positive and negative effects they have on the skin.

Keeping with the theme of love and relationships, to further your understanding of skin care you should begin to view label reading and cosmetic ingredients like you would when you evaluate a potential mate.

Whether we are willing to admit it or not, when we meet or see someone who may become a potential "partner," we size them up. Whether it be during a split-second first impression, while forming a friendship, or dating, we are trying to find out what this person is made of. What is their potential to give us what we are looking for in a mate? Be it love, companionship, security, commitment, or trust, there is something we seek in them. Of course in relationships, they are doing the same to us. However, it's not so unlike shopping for skin care except you are giving your hard earned cash, instead of your heart, in exchange for what you need that product to do for you. By better understanding what your skin care products are made of, you can better gauge their potential to do whatever it is you are asking them to. This will save you time and money. Just like the proper evaluation of a mate will save you from heartache!

It's a lot easier with products, because manufacturers are required to list what they are made of. Can you imagine how much easier dating would be if a potential mate had to list what they had under the hood? How great would it be if you were at a nightclub or event and they had to present you with a card (or picture) that listed all of their qualities, both good and bad, before you would give them the time of day? That would definitely change the dating landscape!

Fortunately, in the land of cosmetics there are several great lists: cosmetic Ingredient encyclopedias like <u>A Consumer's Dictionary of Cosmetic Ingredients</u> by Ruth Winter M.S., and <u>Don't Go to the Cosmetic Counter Without Me</u> by Paula Begoun, are indispensable if you would like a complete resource. I have used them, personally and professionally, for many years.

There is quite a bit of controversy over cosmetic ingredients' link to cancer. Parabens, sulfates, and petrochemicals like mineral oil being the most commonly discussed. There is little research being done, and what evidence there is falls on both sides of the debate. Where it does or does not, however, is less relevant than the fact that manufacturers do not need to use questionable ingredients. They do so because they are inexpensive and easily obtained, and because companies (and the FDA) claim they are safe in small amounts. Since we use cosmetics so often, it is important to know what we are putting on our skin, and the effects accumulated over a lifetime. There are alternatives, manufacturers do not have to use potentially harmful ingredients. The only way companies will change their formulations is through consumer awareness and a demand for higher quality, safe, effective cosmetics.

Until then, you can read labels and evaluate products, yourself. For a beginner's understanding of product ingredients, we will break them down into six categories. Many ingredients can be both a "Functional" (Inactive) or "Performance" (Active) agent, depending on what it's intended to do. For example, water can be a carrier for ingredients, and a hydrator for the skin (as in a toner). Here are the categories, what they do, and some of the top ones you want to Love, Like, or Leave (in alphabetical order):

PRODUCT CATEGORIES

Binders, Fillers, and Carriers
Substances that help the ingredients mix, hold them together, provide texture of product.

Love: Aloe Vera Gel, Corn Starch, Glycerin, Water.

Like: Cellulose, Gelatin, Glucose, Kaolin, Mica, Oat, Pectin, Polysorbates, Rice, Silica, Sodium Hyaluronate.

Leave: Dioxane (PEG and those ending in '-eth' and '-oxynol'), Gluten, Nylon, Polyacrylamide, Stearalkonium Chloride, Talc, Vinyl.

Emollients and Humectants

Fatty substances (like oils,) that moisturize, and ingredients that draw hydration to the surface of the skin (emollients usually end in '-ate').

Love: Aloe Vera Gel, Canola, Ceramides, Glycerin, Hylauronic Acid, Jojoba esters, Safflower, Sodium PCA, Sunflower, Water.

Like: Algae extracts, Allantoin, Caprylyl Glycol EHG, Castor Oil, Cocoa Butter, Coconut Oil, Palm, and Olive Oils, Sorbitol, Sugars: Fructose, Glucose, Sucrose, Seaweed, Shea Butter. Fatty Acids: capric, caprylic, lauric, myristic, oleic, palmitic, and stearic.

Leave: Lanolin, Liquid Paraffin, Mineral Oil, Petrolatum, Propylene Glycol, Petroleum, Prefixes: Benzyl-, Butyl-, Cetearyl-, Cetyl-, Glyceryl-, Isopropyl-, Myristyl-, or Stearyl-.

Cosmeceuticals

Ingredients intended to improve the health and appearance of skin.

Love: Vitamins A, B, C, D, E, F, H, & K. Amino acids and proteins, Azulen, Beta and Poly Glucans and Glycoproteins from Yeast, Ferulic Acid, all Peptides, Retinol.

Like: Alpha-Lipoic Acid, Caffeine, CoEnyme Q-10 (CoQ-10), Green Tea, Glycation, Herbal extracts, Hydroxy Acid, Idebenone, Sirtuins, Tissue Respiratory Factor (TRF), Turmeric.

Leave: None

Surfactants

Ingredients that go underneath dirt and oil and lift debris from skin (soaps and detergents). Can also include Categories 1 and 2.

Love: Saponaria Extract, Saponin,

Like: Castile, Cocamidopropyl Betaine.

Leave: Fluoro-, PEG's, Poloxamer, Sodium Lauryl / Laureth Sulfate.

Preservatives

Substances that fight bacteria and keep the product stable over time.

Love: Antioxidants A, C, and E (tocopherols), Citric Acid, Fructose, Menthol, Tea Tree Oil.

Like: Benzoic acid, Benzylalcohol-, DHA, Potassium Sorbate, Sodium Benzoate.

Leave: Butyl, Ethyl, Methyl, and Propyl, Parabens, Diazolidinyl, Formaldehyde (Quanternium-15 and DMDM hydantoin), Imidazolidinyl Urea, Phenoxyethanol, Thimerosal, Urea.

Color and Fragrance

Give products their appearance and scent.

Love: Annatto, Beet, Chromium oxide, Iron oxide, Saffron, Titanium dioxide, Zinc oxide.

Like: Barium Sulfate, Beta Carotene, Chlorophyll, Limonene, Linalool, Magnesium, Mica, Silica.

Leave: Any Synthetic Colors: "F&DC No.'s and D&C No.'s," and "Lakes," Any Synthetic "Fragrance," Cochineal, Ethylene Oxide, Phthalates (DHP, DBP5, DEHP), Tartrazine.

Miscellaneous

Multiple categories.

Buffers: Adjust the pH of a product: Alkanolamines, Ammonium Bicarbonate, Calcium Carbonate, Citric and Tartaric Acid.

Questionable: Ammonium Lauryl Sulfate, Butylene Glycol, Cetyl Alcohol, Dimethicone, Polyvinyl Acetate, Silicones.

Leave: Aluminum Salts, Diethanolamine (DEA), Monoethanolamine (MEA), Nitrates, PABA, Styrene, Tri-ethanolamine (TEA).

Love Note: Many product companies create synthetic ingredients or a variant of another company's ingredient and give it a complicated name that no one is familiar with, to sneak things in or to protect their own formulations. I tend to stay away from these ingredients. This is where a cosmetic dictionary can help you figure out what it is a variation of.

The FDA requires foods and cosmetics to list all ingredients based on the amount of the ingredient it contains, from the greatest amount listed first, to the least amount listed last. Keep in mind, not all cosmetics are 100% "natural" (meaning from a plant or animal source versus synthetically produced). Products may contain a minute amount of these ingredients that companies aren't even required to list, but still do. These would be the last several ingredients listed. www.CosDNA.com is an awesome database where you can enter a product by name, and it displays the ingredient list, the category of ingredient, and safety rating!

Once you get a general idea of what products are made of, you can quickly look at the label and size up its potential to give your skin what it needs. You want to look for the desired ingredients high on the list. Once you know ingredients that are red flags, you can scan your labels for them, and make an educated decision for yourself.

A product's ingredient list is your opportunity to determine what it can do for you, so don't miss this chance. When you are able to evaluate the majority of ingredients in your products (or at least what category they are from) you will know whether to love it, like it, or leave it on the shelf.

Long and Short Term Product Commitments

How long should you use a product before you know it's working or making a difference? I believe if a product works, it works right away. You should begin to see an improvement, even if it's slight, from the first or second use. Then, the improvements should continue with regular use, or over the next six weeks to three months. The right product will keep your skin looking good.

If you don't see any difference at all, STOP using it. I have mentioned this previously, but it's worth revisiting. Products (like relationships) should not be some huge Enigma: Is it working? What is it doing? Should I keep using it? The only products that deserve to be on your face are the ones that are working for it. Don't fall for a product company's verbiage such as, "Could see results in as little as 6-12 weeks," because this is their way of getting you to use it up before you decide whether it did anything or not! That would be like saying, "Eat this entire meal before you decide if it tastes good."

I am not saying products can give you all the results you want in one use. It took time to get your skin into whatever condition you are addressing, therefore it will take time to get it out. Still, you should be able to wake up each morning after a product has been on your face and say, "My skin does look better than it did before I went to bed." After a long day, say, "I really liked how that product made my skin feel, or helped condition all day." If you can't, send it back!

The same holds true for adverse reactions to a product. The old excuses, "It may worsen the condition before it starts to improve it" and "It's getting rid of toxins and cleaning out your pores" are grossly misused, as well. This is also a company's way of saying, "If you break out, it's your skin's fault, not ours." If this idea of "your skin getting worse before it gets better" is ever true, it should happen briefly, such as 1-2 days, then begin to improve. If it lasts longer than that, it is just aggravating the condition you were trying to treat.

Do you need to be exclusive to one skin care line? No, you can have a variety of brands in your product arsenal. Only use one entire line if each product in the line is working for you. Likewise, it's best to add one new product into to your regimen at a time, to see how your skin responds to it. If you change all your products and you react adversely, it's likely you will stop using them all. This applies to DIY recipes, makeup, or anything new.

Don't give products free reign on your face! Just like you shouldn't give a partner free reign in your life. Make them prove themselves to you (and your skin), by doing what they say they will do.

Love Lesson #7

What's Your Type?

Studies show that most women incorrectly identify their skin type and home care regimen. Are you unsure what type of skin you have and if you are choosing the right products for it? You may be selecting ones that are incompatible for you. It's time to understand your skin like a professional and find the best matches for it. Let's work up a profile of your skin to find its type. These are the topics and questions I would discuss with you during a skin care consultation, before a treatment, or with a product selection. It's important to know your skin, and to recognize what improvements you want to see in it.

SKIN SELF ASSESSMENT

1. Describe Your Skin

Finish the following sentence either mentally, orally, or written down on a separate piece of paper: My skin is: _____. Try to be detailed. Need some help? Here are a few common examples:

•My skin is dry on my cheeks and oily on my forehead, nose, and chin.

•Breakouts occur regularly and for no specific reason.

•Breakouts occur before or during my menstrual cycle.

•My skin has significant signs of aging and loss of elasticity.

•My skin is very sensitive and has redness and broken capillaries.

•I have large pores, many of which are congested.

•My skin is fairly decent and I would like to keep it that way.

•My skin is past the point of no return.

•I have discoloration and uneven skin tone.

•My skin is rough textured and I would like it to be smoother and glowing.

2. Improvements

Next, state what improvements you would like to see in your skin. Again, be detailed: "I want my skin to be _____."

Common improvements could be: firmer, younger, smoother, cleaner, more hydrated, even-toned, or clearer with fewer breakouts.

3. Oil Production

Skin care professionals use the amount of oil your skin produces and when it produces it to determine your skin type. How many hours after you wash your face do you see any trace of oil on your skin?

Less than 1 hour to 2 hours later (Oily or Acneic).

Between 2-3 hours later (Oily to Combination).

Between 3-5 hours later (Combination to Normal).

Between 5-7 hours later (Normal or Pre-Aging).

No oil production on skin (Dry or Mature).

4. Sensitivity

Have you ever had a reaction to a product or cosmetic such as redness, itching, burning, rash, or hives?

Yes, frequently (Sensitive / Reactive).

Yes, but rarely (Normal to Sensitive).

No, I have never had a reaction (Non-Reactive).

Sometimes with love, you need to do a little stalking. Let's dig deeper and find more about what your skin is up to. This will be the final determination to identify your type. Your skin is complex and may have multiple types, depending on the physiological function. For example, you could have Oily skin, with no sensitivities, but premature aging. You could have normal oil production, but be highly sensitive. I currently have premature aging, normal to dry skin, with no sensitivities. Six months ago I had premature aging, oily skin, with sensitivities. Get the picture? Once you know your current profile, you can choose the products and treatments to address each function specifically.

Match your answers from the four previous questions to the ones below. Go through each of the following categories and find the statements that most closely match yours. Then, we will customize your type!

Normal Skin

Whose skin is "normal?" Not many of ours! It's more normal to have skin concerns than it is to not have them, but the term "normal" refers to standard, healthy functions; everything is operating as it should be. The goal for normal skin is maintenance. If any aspect of your skin is functioning properly, the statement(s) in the matching category will apply:

Common Descriptions for Normal Skin (Question 1):

I don't have many concerns with my skin. I've always had "good" skin.

I use soap and water, and sometimes don't wash my face at all.

Improvements (Question 2):

I would like to keep my skin looking healthy.

I would like a healthy "glow."

Oil Production (Question 3):

I see oil between 5-7 hours after cleansing or none at all.

Sensitivity (Question 4):

I have no reactions to products or cosmetics.

Combination Skin

Indicates you have multiple areas on your face functioning differently, at the same time. It does not mean your skin is dry one day, then oily the next. It means your skin is dry and oily on the same day! It doesn't just have to be oily and dry, either. It can be any of the skin types, on multiple areas of your face. The goal for combination skin is balance. If any of your skin's functions are the combination type, the statement(s) in the matching category will apply:

Common Descriptions for Combination Skin:

I have dry patches on my cheeks and oily patches on my forehead, nose, and chin.

Products applied all over my face work in some areas, and not in others.

I often need to change the products I am using, and still may not see any difference.

If I have a breakout, it is usually in the T-Zone area.

I can never figure out if I am using the right products!

Improvements:

I would like smoother, clearer skin all over.

I would like less redness and more even tone.

I need one product for multiple concerns.

Oil Production:

I see oil on certain areas of my face between 2-5 hours after cleansing, it varies.

Sensitivity:

Yes, I have sensitivity to products and cosmetics, but I never know to what, or when it will occur.

Oily Skin

I often found if a client has any oil production at all, they think they have oily skin and use products to "dry out" the skin, or that are "Oil-Free." True oily skin means there is an overproduction of oil from the sebaceous (oil) glands. It is normal to have oil production, just not one or two hours after cleansing. The goal for oily skin is less activity. If your skin is overproducing sebum (oil), then the following statements will match yours:

Common Descriptions for Oily Skin:

I have oil shine over my entire face.

I need to blot my skin throughout the day.

I have a thicker, bumpy, textured skin.

I have large pores all over.

Improvements:

I would like less shine and smaller pores.

I want smoother, finer textured skin.

Oil Production:

I see oil production less than one hour and up to two hours after cleansing.

Sensitivity:

I could probably put anything on my skin without a reaction. It's very tough.

Acneic Skin

If you have acneic skin, you can't help but know it. Having an occasional breakout does not mean you have acneic skin. It means you had a breakout. There are four different grades of true acneic skin. Three of them can be treated without a physician. The fourth grade needs some type of prescriptive care. Acneic skin is my specialty and I will offer a large amount of detailed information on this skin type in its corresponding Love Lesson. The goal for acneic skin is improved resistance.

Common Descriptions for Acneic Skin:

I have 5-10 regular to severe blemishes on most areas of my face.

Breakouts occur either with my menstrual cycle or consistently. Wasn't this supposed to stop after puberty?

Just when I think I've gotten things under control, or a product is working, I have another breakout.

Nothing seems to clear up my skin.

Improvements:

No more acne!

Clearer, even-toned, smoother, deep-clean skin.

I want to know what it's like to not worry about having a breakout.

Oil Production:

I see oil between 2-3 hours after cleansing.

Sensitivity:

It seems like everything I use causes a breakout or irritation of some kind.

Reactive / Sensitive Skin

This skin type is easily misunderstood. True sensitive skin has reactions that can be considered "allergic" in nature, meaning that irritants cause swelling, itching, hives, bumps, scaling, or redness. Sensitive skin does not mean that a product was not compatible for your skin. There are individuals who cannot put anything on their face, including water. This is the most extreme form of sensitivity. The goal for this fragile skin type is strengthening. If you have reactive / sensitive skin, the following statements will resemble yours:

Common Descriptions for Sensitive Skin:

Many products I use cause irritation.

I am afraid to try new products; I use very basic cleanser and moisturizer that my dermatologist recommended.

I've given up on skin care.

I often have peeling, flaking, and red areas on my face.

Improvements:

I would like to be able to use skin care products without worrying what reaction I may have.

I would like to reduce the redness in my skin.

I wish I could go without wearing heavy concealer and foundation, which also tend to irritate my skin.

Oil Production:

I can see oil production on my skin anywhere between 1-7 hours after cleansing. It varies, and usually corresponds with a flare-up.

Sensitivity:

You're talking to the Queen / King of sensitive skin. Everything irritates it.

Prematurely Aging Skin

This is the polite way of saying, "You've put your skin through Hell, and it shows." Don't beat yourself up about it, the damage has been done, and it can be undone. You've just got to come to terms with the fact that you will have to make some lifestyle changes, and put in some work. The damage didn't happen to anyone's skin in one day, and it can't be reversed in one day either. The goal for prematurely aging skin is repair and regeneration. If you are in need of some anti-aging, your responses will be similar to the following:

Common Descriptions for Prematurely Aging Skin:

I have had a great deal of sun exposure over the years, including indoor tanning.

I have areas of darker pigmentation and spots on my face.

I have lines and loss of firmness in multiple areas.

My skin feels rough in texture.

I don't know how to reverse the aging process.

Improvements:

I would like: firmer, plumper, more even toned skin.

I would like to lessen the lines and discontinue the formation of new ones.

I want supermodel skin. I am still young enough!

Oil Production:

I see a small amount of oil, later in the day.

I do still have breakouts, but not consistently.

Sensitivity:

I do not have any sensitivities to speak of. My skin seems rather dull and lifeless.

Dry and Mature Skin

These two types are categorized together because they have one thing in common: the lack of oil production. You can be young and have dry skin. You can be older and still have oily skin. Mature / dry skin means you are at the point where your sebaceous glands are no longer producing any oil. The goal for dry and mature skin types is stimulation of oil production, increased metabolism, and protection. If your skin isn't producing oil, it is dry and your statements will be comparable to the following:

Common Descriptions for Dry and Mature Skin:

My skin feels tight or itchy. It often peels or flakes.

My skin is thin, delicate or crepe-like.

I have used a product or medication that caused me to have dry skin.

It never seems like I can moisturize enough.

I am postmenopausal or no longer have estrogen production.

I have loss of firmness and sagging in areas of my face and neck.

I have deep lines and wrinkles.

I feel I am past the point of reversing the aging process and/or I am considering plastic surgery.

Improvements:

What improvements wouldn't I like to see?

I would like to look more rested, and youthful again.

I want softer, healthier, glowing skin.

Oil Production:

I NEVER see oil on my skin.

Sensitivity:

Some products do cause itching, redness, and peeling or flaking of my skin, especially pigmented cosmetics. Many products seem too harsh for my skin.

Your Custom Type

Next, use your answers from questions 1-4 to identify your type. Your skin has an overall type—choose the type that most resembles your responses from (Questions 1 and 2) Descriptions and Improvements. Your skin's Oil Production (Question 3), has a type and so does your Sensitivity

Level (Question 4). These are your subtypes. You may have anywhere from one type, or a combination of three different types.

Now you can follow the recommendations for your skin type and subtypes (if applicable) in each of the proceeding Love Lessons to better understand your skin, create your personalized skin care regimen, and choose the right products and treatments for it. If you have multiple skin types, remember—your skin can change daily, or during any hormonal or physiological changes in your body. I recommend assessing your skin on a daily basis and using the products for that skin type. I will continue to expand on this as we progress. Next, let's learn about each of the steps that should be part of your skin care rituals, and then what your skin type needs.

Love Lesson #8

Skin Care Rituals

Bondage, anyone? All relationships need a little variety to keep things interesting, even your skin! Does trying something new scare you, or do you love the thrill of the new and unknown? It doesn't matter where your comfort zone is at, you've got to get out of it and try new things in your routine if you are going to get skin care satisfaction!

When it comes to daily skin care routines, I find there are two types of women: those that are okay using several products on their skin, morning and night, and those who are not. Women who are accustomed to using multiple products usually have an easier time making changes to their daily routine and trying new things. The "soap and water, maybe a moisturizer" friends can be more resistant to changes in their regimens and trying new products. I do believe the women in the later group may embrace differences in their skin care rituals if they were to go out of their comfort zone a bit more. In contrast, if you are already using many products, you might be tired of the same drill day after day, and could use something new and exciting, too.

Skin care can be fun and sexy, if you know what to do, and when! The following Love Lessons detail the steps in a full skin care regimen and how to do it like the pros. (Sorry, it doesn't include whips and chains...but, at least the bondage comment got you thinking!) Here are the steps for your morning and evening rituals:

MORNING

1. Cleanse
2. Exfoliate (Shower only. Frequency: per skin type)
3. Tone (First step after showering)
4. Serum
5. Moisturize
6. Protect
7. Eye / Lip
8. Makeup

EVENING

9. Double Cleanse (per skin type)
10. Tone
11. Serum
12. Moisturize
13. Eye / Lip

WEEKLY

Masque and deep exfoliant 1-2 times as directed per skin type.

DRESS YOUR FACE

Do you already have difficulty remembering what order to apply your products during your AM & PM regimens? I've come up with another analogy to help you remember them: Apply products to your face like you dress your body, day and night. The idea is that the clothes in your wardrobe serve a similar purpose as the products in your skin care routine, and in the same order.

AM after you shower (Cleanse) you put on:

Body mist or perfume (Tone)

Undergarments (Serum)

Clothes (Moisturizer)

Overcoat (Protection / SPF)

Accessories (Eyes / Lips & Makeup)

You wouldn't put your bra and panties over your clothing, would you? Likewise, you wouldn't put your serum on top of your moisturizer. You need support under them, not on top. You wouldn't go outside without clothing (Moisturizer), or not wear a coat on a cold day (SPF)? What about your purse or jewelry (Eye / Lip & Makeup)? Layer them from what you want closest to your skin, first—to what you want protecting you, last. I hope this helps you keep them straight.

PM after you bathe (Cleanse) you wear:

Body mist (just pretend)! (Tone)

Sleep undergarments (Serum)

Pajamas (Moisturizer)

Slippers! (Eyes / Lips)

Sorry, no sleeping in the nude when it comes to skin care! To remember the order, you can use a permanent marker to write the number of their AM and PM order on the lid of the products. If you are not currently doing any of the aforementioned steps, your skin may be missing out on more than you think. The next Love Lessons will teach you how to do these steps like a pro, and why you must include them in your routine to maintain a healthy love life with your skin.

If all of these steps seem like too much, that's okay. Do the best you can. Your skin will respond to what you do for it, far better than your doing nothing at all. Less is not more, when it comes to skin care. Less is less! I don't know who started the "Less is more" rumor, but it isn't true. Your skin needs all the steps in the daily rituals. It can't use what you don't give it, and it surely can't get it for itself. This holds true, as long as what you are putting on (and in) your body is good for it.

Love Note: I've listed my top product recommendations for each skin type in the following Love Lessons. When possible, I've provided the company's website, but you will still have to search for the product by name. Included are recommendations from drugstore through prescription grades. As I've previously mentioned, I cannot possibly research every product from every company on the market. I have spent years, poring over as many as I could, so you don't have to. If I do not list it, and it is a well known brand, chances are it's not "Love Your Skin approved," meaning it doesn't match the criteria included in the book. There were many products I wanted to recommend, but didn't, due to the additives. Please note: The products and prices listed are subject to change, as they represent what the company provided at the time this edition was published.

I encourage you to use the information I've given you when reading labels to evaluate whether a product can give you what you're looking for. If you want to submit a product you love, send me an email and if it meets the LYS criteria, I may include it in upcoming editions. LoveYourSkin@NicciLeigh.com

Many of the products recommended can be bought at a local retailer, spa, or specialty shop. If you don't know where to find what you're looking for, check their website- it may very well list their locations.

Love Lesson #9

Cleanse

Go to bed with your makeup on? Never! We all know this is the #1 Cardinal Sin when it comes to skin. Let me tell you why, and how to do it right—Love Your Skin style. I have recommended this slight adjustment to many of my clients and they have seen a dramatic improvement in their skin, especially if they have oily, blemished, or acne prone skin.

PM Cleanse: This is the most important time to wash up, because throughout the day, your face has been front and center for everything the world has dished out: dirt, bacteria, oil, pollution, dead skin cells shed on a daily basis, and more. While you sleep, your skin decides what it needs to do in accordance to what's on it. So, get that junk off of it!

How to Cleanse Like a Pro — Double Cleanse: Use a more powerful cleanser at night than you would in the morning. Choose one that foams or lathers, preferably non-soap based. Place the cleanser on your hands with water and LIGHTLY cleanse your face—then rinse. Here's the expert tip: Cleanse again! Get another dime to nickel sized amount, lather and apply. This time, massage the cleanser DEEPER into all areas. Use your fingertips and really work that cleanser into every nook and cranny of your face: the sides of your nose, inner cheeks, the center of your chin, your full cheeks and forehead. Then rinse. If you do this, you will have cleaner pores, fewer breakouts, and healthier skin. Here's why: The first cleanse removes the top layer of oil, dirt, makeup, and anything else on the surface. If you were to try to deep cleanse your face on the first cleanse (which you may be doing now), it has the opposite effect and pushes the debris further down into your pores, leaving them clogged and prone to a breakout. Get rid of it first by gently lifting it off with the first cleanse, then go back for a second cleanse and work the product deeper into the pores, purifying them fully on this round.

Typically, we are in such a hurry when we wash our face at night that we do a quick "once over," then rinse. The problem is that, over time, the debris that's left on your skin builds up in your pores, leaving your skin busy at night trying to push it out instead of resting and regenerating those pretty little cells. Double cleanse in the PM!

Side note about eye makeup remover: You should use a product that is gentle, non drying, non-soap based to remove eye makeup either before or after your cleanse. Some women prefer a cream based product to break the makeup down, and wipe it away. Sometimes I even use my eye cream or a richer face cream. There is really no way to get around using eye makeup remover if you wear heavy mascara or liner.

AM Cleanse Like a Pro: If you shower in the morning, wash your face LAST, after you have rinsed your conditioner out. Hair conditioner has no place on your face. It contains oils, waxes, and other ingredients that are not face friendly. When you tip your head back and rinse your hair, by default, the conditioner rinses down onto the skin around your hairline, cheeks, forehead and chin. This is the number one cause of forehead and cheek breakouts that have a small, raised, bumpy texture. Heavy conditioners are designed to repair all the terrible things we do to our hair, and will clog the pores on your face if your skin is prone to breakouts. (If you change this one step in your routine you will see a drastic difference. If you are not prone to breakouts, you will not see much of a change, but you still don't want conditioner on your face.)

So, wash your face last when showering. You can use a more gentle cleanser in the morning than you do in the evening (like a cream, milk, or lotion) since you don't have much to wash away. If you have oily or acneic skin, you may want to stick with the stronger cleanser to remove oil production that occurred at night. If you don't shower in the morning, still do the light cleanse, and do the double cleanse when you shower in the evening. Commit to cleansing properly and you will have a long term healthy relationship with your skin.

Types of Cleansers

Note to our "soap and water" friends-Soaps, on average, have a pH of 9-10, which is much too alkaline for your skin which has a natural pH of 5.5 (neutral is 7). It will over-dry your skin and disturb its protective outer layer: the acid mantle. Try using a cleanser tailored for your skin type (recommendations still to come).

Gel: Creates lather, usually a deep cleanse, best for oily and acneic skin types. Look for non-soap based gel cleansers, as soaps and sulfates are too harsh for your face.

Lotion: These cleansers look like a lotion or have a milky consistency, but gently lather when water is added to them and applied to the face. Best for combination and non-reactive "normal" skin types.

Cream: Only use if you have dry, mature, or sensitive, non-acneic skin. They usually do not produce a lather and can be used with or without water. Some cleansers for extremely dry or sensitive skin are removed with a tissue or damp washcloth. As stated before, there are people who are even sensitive to water.

Oil: Yes, oil cleanses! Oil cleansers have been used very successfully for acneic—especially cystic—skin types. Here's why: oil is attracted to oil. It is able to loosen hard oil deposits deep within the pores and pull them loose. Oil and water molecules have "tails" on them which are able to attach to other receptive oil and water molecules. Oil cleansers are a popular product in Europe, and usually followed by a second cleanser. When using an oil cleanser you first apply the oil to DRY skin (no water) and massage lightly, then use a clean washcloth and very warm water to remove. I've included a DIY recipe and recommendations for you in upcoming chapters. Oil cleansers can be beneficial to all skin types, you will have to try it and see if it is right for your skin.

Whatever you do, don't commit the #1 Cardinal Sin and skip a cleanse! Your skin deserves better.

CLEANSER RECOMMENDATIONS BY SKIN TYPE

All Skin Types

Mineral Face Cleanser (powder) $8 www.eyeslipsface.com

Rosa Centifolia Cleansing Gel $32 www.RenSkincare.com

Precleanse (oil cleanser) $35 www.dermalogica.com

Start Up (Exfoliating Face Wash)$12.75, Olive Oil Bar-Soaps $2.99-3.99 www.kissmyface.com

Streetwise Gentle Antioxidant Face Wash $21 www.OricoLondon.com

Keys Island Rx Foaming Facial Cleanser $16.95 www.keys-soap.com

Combination Skin

Special Cleansing Gel (deep clean w/o drying) $34
www.dermalogica.com

Neutrogena® Naturals Fresh Cleansing + Makeup Remover $7.49 www.neutrogena.com

Balancing Cleansing Emulsion $36
www.BeingTrue.com

Mayblosssom T-Zone Control Cleansing Gel $32
www.RenSkincare.com

Clean For A Day (Creamy Face Cleanser) $12.75
www.kissmyface.com

Oily Skin

HY-ÖL and Combination Phytoactive (2 part oil and herbal cleanse) $28 www.Babor.com

Mint Soufflé $17 www.RayaSpa.com Call to order.

Neutrogena® Naturals Purifying Cleanser $7.49
www.neutrogena.com

DDF Glycolic 5% Exfoliating Wash $39
www.ddfskincare.com

ClearCalm 3 Clarifying Clay Cleanser $32
www.RenSkincare.com

Aloe Cleansing Gel $14-28.00 www.naturopathica.com

Acneic Skin (see Oily Skin)

Purifying Gel Cleanser (adult) $10 www.burtsbees.com

Cleansing Gel and Tonic 2 in 1 $36 www.Babor.com

Purifying Glycolic Cleanser $36 www.BeingTrue.com

DDF Blemish Foaming Cleanser $39
www.ddfskincare.com

Neutrogena® Naturals Acne Cream Cleanser $8.49
www.neutrogena.com

In the Clear $26 www.purminerals.com

Anti-Blemish Facial Wash $22 www.BelliSkincare.com

Sensitive / Reactive Skin

Azulen Cleansing Milk $16 (healing, used with or without water) www.RayaSpa.com Call to order.

UltraCalming Cleanser (soothing) $34
www.dermalogica.com

Sensitive Facial Cleanser (moisturizing and soothing)
$10 www.burtsbees.com

Sensitive Skin Cleanser $45.50 (water activated oil)
www.bioelements.com

DDF Sensitive Skin Cleansing Gel $39
www.ddfskincare.com

Hydra-Calm Cleansing Milk and Gel $32
www.RenSkincare.com

Chamomile Cleansing Milk $28
www.naturopathica.com

Prematurely Aging Skin

Silky Cleanser (refining) $16 www.RayaSpa.com

Tri Active Cleanse (brightens) $38
www.dermalogica.com

Radiance Facial Cleanser (cell turnover) $10
www.burtsbees.com

DDF Brightening Cleanser (AHA & BHA) $39
www.ddfskincare.com

Micro Polish Cleanser $30 www.RenSkincare.com

Dry / Mature Skin

SkinLogics® Essential Cleansing Cream (multivitamin)
$21 www.beauticontrol.com

Intense Hydration Cream Cleanser $10
www.burtsbees.com

Baborganic Glacier Cleansing Milk $34
www.Babor.com

Restoring Deep Cleanser (oil) $36 www.BeingTrue.com

Chamomile Cleansing Milk $16 www.RayaSpa.com

Ultra Moisture Cleansing Milk $32
www.RenSkincare.com

Eye Makeup Removers

Eye Make-up Remover $12.95 www.RayaSpa.com

Simple brand Eye Makeup Remover $7.29 (drugstores)

SkinLogics® Lash Enhancing Eye Makeup Remover $12 www.BeautiControl.com

Pure Comfort™ Eye Makeup Remover $18 www.Aveda.com

Purity Cleansing Balm $48 www.RenSkincare.com

Streetwise Hydrating Make-up Remover for Face and Eyes $25 www.OricoLondon.com

Love Lesson #10

Tone

Think of toning as an extension of your cleanse, like the final step in washing your face. Before we go any further, let's make a distinction between a toner and an astringent. An astringent contains alcohol, a toner does not. Alcohol dries the skin and kills bacteria. Therefore, you should only use a product containing alcohol over an area of breakouts, or to spot treat a pimple. If you are using an astringent all over your face because you have oily skin, you are just drying it out, so it thinks it needs to make MORE oil to moisturize your face! Toners, on the other hand, can be used morning and night, or anytime you wash your face. They: 1. Remove traces of cleanser and all the other stuff you were trying to wash away. 2. Hydrate the skin. 3. Restore your skin's pH balance. (This is the natural acidity (sour / bitter) or alkalinity (salty / sweet) of your skin.) The normal pH of the skin is between 4.5-6.5 with the middle of the pH scale being 7—below 7 is acidic, above is alkaline. Here's the catch: in order for a cleanser to work (remove debris) it needs to be slightly more acidic or alkaline than your skin. Otherwise, it won't do anything. The pH of a cleanser depends on the type of cleanser that it is, and the skin type it is made for. Gels are typically more acidic, and lotions, milks, and creams more alkaline. Alkaline products can be drying, while acidic ones can irritate. After cleansing, a toner will restore your skin to its balanced pH. A balanced pH leads to less reactive skin, meaning less oil, less sensitivity—essentially, more well-behaved skin!

How to Tone and When: You can either wipe or mist your toner. Tone in the morning and evening. Wipe: Saturate a cotton pad and lightly wipe or pat in an upward motion. Mist: Buy a small spray bottle and mix half toner, half distilled water, and mist your face. (This method balances pH and hydrates, but does not remove traces of cleanser and other un-wanteds.) I like to spray my toner into the palm of my hand and apply almost like a serum. This is great when your skin needs extra hydration.

I've observed what I'll call the "Toner Epidemic," or the lack thereof, in skin care regimens. I think this may be because there are so few toners available at the drugstore level; the ones that are available contain alcohol, and many of us have had negative experiences with "astringents" that burned or dried out our skin. There are many great toners out there, and it's easy to make your own (See DIY Skin Care). So please don't skip the toner, it is a more important part of a healthy skin relationship than people give it credit for. Quite often when women add a toner to their skin care regimen, they see a HUGE improvement in their skin, over all.

TONER RECOMMENDATIONS BY SKIN TYPE

All Skin Types

Aloe-Cucumber Astringent (non alcohol) $15.50 www.RayaSpa.com Call to order.

Baborganic Pure Energizing Skin Water $34 www.Babor.com

Multiactive Toner $32 www.dermalogica.com

Tonic Moisture Mist $28 www.RenSkinCare.com

Balancing Act Facial Toner $12.75 www.kissmyface.com

Combination Skin

Equalizer $29 www.bioelements.com

Simple brand Soothing Facial Toner $7.29 Available at most drug and retail stores.

Chamomile Toner $14.95-40.00 www.Vasseurskincare.com

Deep Pore Freshener (also suitable for oily and Acneic skin types) $16.50 www.lbri.com

Oily Skin

Menthol Astringent $15.50 www.RayaSpa.com

Equalizing Toner (alpha hydroxy acid (AHA), pore minimizing) $30 www.skinceuticals.com

Essential Clarifying Tonic $31 www.BeingTrue.com

Papaya Enzyme Toner $14-95-40.00 www.Vasseurskincare.com

Acneic Skin

Camphor Astringent (AHA) $15.50, Ginseng Astringent (AHA, dries breakouts, non-irritating) $16 www.RayaSpa.com

Conditioning Solution (AHA & beta hydroxy acid BHA) $30 www.skinceuticals.com

Concentrated Balancing Toner $32.95 www.Sukiskincare.com

Clarifying Toning Lotion $28 www.RenSkincare.com

Sensitive / Reactive Skin

Aloe-Cucumber Astringent (non-alcohol, mild, and healing) $15.50 www.RayaSpa.com

UltaCalming Mist (healing) $32 www.Dermalogica.com

SkinLogics® Sensitive Rinse and Restore Tonic $22 www.Beauticontrol.com

Essential Soothing Tonic $31 www.BeingTrue.com

Gentle Freshener $16.50 www.lbri.com

Prematurely Aging Skin

Essential-C Toner $28 www.Murad.com

Ginseng Astringent Toner (non-alcohol, AHA, oxygenates) Use once a day or dilute. $16 www.RayaSpa.com

Antioxidant Hydramist $38 www.Dermalogica.com

Concentrated Nourishing Toner $29.95 www.Sukiskincare.com

Dry / Mature Skin

Power Peptide (firming) $39 www.bioelements.com

Rose Toning Lotion (non-alcohol) $30 www.babor.com

glō minerals Moist Hydration Mist $18 www.gloprofessional.com

Lavender Honey Balancing Mist, & Rose Geranium Soothing Mist $28 www.naturopathica.com

Love Lesson #11

Exfoliate

Oh...where do we begin? Exfoliation is the one step that gives you the most opportunity to see a difference in your skin. Exfoliating is like dusting a coffee table. After you wipe away all the dust that's built up, the beautiful wood grain is visible and shining again. Seems self explanatory, right? Well, exfoliating is easily underestimated because there are many ways to do it, more than just an apricot scrub or beads in your cleanser.

Think of your skin as a brick wall. The layers of bricks are like the layers of your skin cells, and the brick's mortar is like the intercellular glue that holds your cells together. The bricks (cells) on the top often get weathered and worn, and need to be taken off. When you tear down the bricks (cells) on the top, it signals the wall (your skin) to send new bricks (healthy cells) from the bottom. Removing the old bricks lessens the depth of lines, discoloration, and improves skin's overall appearance.

We all build up walls in life, in love, and on our skin. The same way you can't have a healthy relationship with those walls up, neither will your skin be healthy! There's a soft tenderness beneath our wall, and it's time to break them down to get to it! How are we best going to do it?

TYPES OF EXFOLIANTS

Scrubs

Scrubs can knock off the top layer of bricks (cells) like a sledge hammer would, depending on how strong they are. Round smooth beads (jojoba, polyurethane, ground nuts, grains and flour) are the most gentle. Square edge exfoliants (sugar and salt crystals) exfoliate with a flat edge, but dissolve when mixed with water. Diamond cut (aluminum oxide) used in microdermabrasion cream scrubs are highly abrasive and most precise. Jagged edged exfoliants (fruit seeds and nut shells) are rough and sometimes irritating. The less sensitive your skin is, the higher level of abrasion it can withstand. There are many experts in the skin care world who believe the jagged edged exfoliants can cause "micro tears" to your skin that produces inflammation; which accelerates aging, and should be avoided. I agree.

The basic idea behind exfoliation is that when you remove layers of cells, your live cell layer beneath them produces "new" cells to replace the ones that were taken. This is ultimately what you want your skin to always be doing: producing new healthy cells. When: Scrubs should only be used in the shower when your skin is softened and warm. Use your exfoliant after you've cleansed, not before.

Rotary Brushes

These would also be considered a "scrub" type of exfoliant. You can find less expensive ones at the drugstore for $15-$20, and more expensive ones online for up to $150. Search "facial brush" on Amazon.com and you will find numerous models available. Is there a significant difference between them? I don't think so. They all remove the surface cell layer, and the ones with "sonic" properties claim to offer a deeper penetration of products as it exfoliates. TEI Spa's UltraCleanse Set $70, includes facial brushes and tools for face and body. www.TeiSpa.com

I think everyone should be using a rotary facial brush. The skin needs daily exfoliation, and these brushes are excellent for regular use. Think of them like a "shave" for your face. Most men shave daily, and when they do, it removes the top several layers, forcing the skin to renew by regenerating fresh cells. They shave the entire lower area of their face and neck, from puberty to old age. Maybe, this is why men seem to age more "gracefully." The areas of the mouth, cheeks, jawline, and neck are the areas that lose elasticity, develop lines, and sag as women age. Whereas these areas on men remain firm and chiseled, late into life. If you took George Clooney and placed him next to a female actor counterpart of his same age, how would you imagine her skin to look in comparison to his, if she had not had any plastic surgery? Would she be given the same accolades for her looks as Clooney would, as they aged? There is a double standard in aging. If you don't believe me, look at a mature man's face: the only lines you will see are on his forehead- the only place he doesn't shave! So, what if women shaved? Is that what I am saying? Yes and no. Men do have thicker skin, more collagen and elastin, more oil glands, and produce oil up to twenty years longer than women do, which can attribute for a slower tendency to show signs of aging. However, we need to be more aggressive in our daily exfoliation. This is, of course, if you do not have any true sensitivities, conditions, or cystic acne. We need to keep those cells turning over. Use a rotary brush daily, in the shower, when your cleanser is on. Don't neglect the shaving areas! Then, use your other exfoliating products throughout the week to exfoliate in more than one way. I do a "double exfoliation" several times per week: I use the rotary brush when my cleanser is on, then I apply an enzyme or hydroxy product afterwards and let it sit while I finish my shower. We can't be afraid of exfoliation. The skin care world has women afraid to use anything "harsh" on their faces, while men are taking a razor to theirs every day! The proper exfoliation does keep cells stimulated. Watch out, Clooney, we're coming for you, baby...

Enzymes

These are made from fruit enzymes like papaya, pineapple, or other natural sources like rice and pumpkin. Enzymes dissolve the bricks (cells). Because they dissolve them, rather than knocking them off with brute force, they are gentler than other exfoliants. Enzyme based products are mostly available in professional grade or high end skin care lines. I do not see many of them available in drugstore or department stores brands. Enzymes are often included in scrubs to make them more effective, and they are the best for sensitive, reactive, and acne prone skin since there is no "rubbing" to cause irritation. ANYONE can use them. When: Enzymes are applied and left to sit on your face, like a masque would. They need steam to work effectively, so use them in the shower. The use of steam is probably why you mainly see them in spa lines. You can leave it on while you shave your legs, and get spa-worthy results!

Chemical Hydroxy Acids

Back to the brick wall analogy, hydroxy acids like alphas and betas dissolve the "mortar" between the bricks—unlocking them so they will lift off the surface. Unlike enzymes which only dissolve the top layer of bricks, hydroxy acids are the most powerful exfoliant we've discussed so far because they unlock that intercellular glue. They are able to penetrate in between the brick layers, removing them. This process can be more irritating than enzymes, depending on the type and strength (percentage) of acid used.

Alphas are more aggressive than betas, and they get more done. Choose which hydroxy is right for you: Alphas (water soluble) like glycolic and lactic are great for premature aging and sun damaged skin, while betas (oil soluble) like salicylic are best for acneic, thicker, oilier types. Alphas work better in higher concentrations and should be in the top three ingredients. Betas work best in lower amounts and used over a longer period. Again, this depends on who you get them from or who applies them. The FDA ruled in

1997 that over-the-counter products must not contain more than 10% acid and no lower of a pH than 3.5. Licensed professionals may sell and apply higher concentrations as previously mentioned in the Love Lesson: "Product Comparisons."

When: Depending on your skin type, use alpha or beta hydroxy acids in cleansers, toners, as home peels, in moisturizers and masks. For Anti-Aging: gradually increase the use of any form of alpha (not beta) hydroxy product from two times per week up to as often as twice a day. For Acneic Skin: slowly incorporate products that contain them (beta and/or alpha), to ensure they are a good match for your skin. You should expect to see smoother, brighter, clearer skin with proper use. Caution: All forms of hydroxy acids can over-dry and irritate skin, causing inflammation. If you experience this, back off of the product and reduce usage by alternating it with non-hydroxy acid products. The inflammation caused by the product is not worth the good it might be doing. The FDA recommends always wearing a SPF of 30 or higher when using Hydroxy acids.

Retinol

This form of vitamin A can be used both as an antioxidant and exfoliant. Retinol can treat a wide range of skin concerns, including acne, skin rejuvenation, pigmentation, reduction of sebum production, improved moisture retention, fine lines and wrinkles. It has frequently been named the number one most important product women should be using in their skin care regimens. It is the most powerful at-home exfoliant you can get. Retinol is able to change the structure of the layers of the epidermis, thus exfoliating the skin, and also responsible for healthy cell functions, which diminish as we age. It can permeate through the skin layers into the dermis, affecting the collagen, elastin, and other tissue fibers there. There are retinol products available from drugstore through physician grades; the stronger the it is, the further reach it has. Over the counter products have only a slight ability to travel, where prescription vitamin A products can penetrate into the blood stream. For this reason, it cannot be used when you are pregnant, nursing, or trying to conceive, as it could harm the baby. It can also affect the skin of your entire body, even if you only apply it to your face. Accutane, an acne medication dermatologists often prescribe to teens, is a form of vitamin A taken internally.

Usage: Many over the counter brands offer products containing vitamin A and retinol, and are safe in these small amounts. You must still adjust the frequency you use them based on how your skin is responding; it is common to experience dry peeling skin several days after application. Use them less if you experience excessive redness and peeling.

Anti-aging: I recommend only using them from fall through spring, never during the summer. Begin use when you are no longer actively outdoors or experiencing daily sun exposure. If you live in a warm climate, you must be diligent with SPF 30 or higher. Start by using them twice a week and gradually increasing as tolerated.

Acneic Skin: use them as directed, and as long as you are seeing an improvement. Vitamin A is oil soluble, so apply it to dry skin, and wait 15-20 min before applying your moisturizer or any other product containing water.

Scarring and Pigmentation: Due to the regenerative and corrective properties of retinoids, they can be used on scars and areas with increased pigmentation. Apply the retinol product directly to the scar, stretch marks, or pigmented area. Wait until the scar or stretch mark has healed completely before applying. Areas like the back of your hands and chest can often have hyper-pigmentation and age spots, and will benefit from retinol, also.

You must use retinol carefully, and under the close supervision of a skin care professional or physician. Because it exposes new skin cells, you must wear an SPF when using a retinol because you run the risk of damaging those new cells you just worked so hard to get.

Chemical Peels

These are powerful exfoliants. Traditional chemical peels are treatments only administered by a skin care professional, aesthetician, nurse, dermatologist, or plastic surgeon. Again, the strength of the peel varies based on who you are receiving it from. Aestheticians can give peels up to 30% concentration, nurses and doctors can administer peels that are up to 70% active ingredients.

Peels do the same things as previously mentioned in the hydroxy acid section, only more aggressively. By taking off the top layers of dead cells, it forces your live cells beneath to produce more and push the new cells forward. As we age, our skin produces fewer of these new cells on its own. Chemical peels stimulate them to do it more often. This is beneficial if you have rough, unevenly textured skin. Fine lines and wrinkles appear less deep when you lift off the unwanted top layers. The look of discoloration lessens when there are fewer pigmented cells visible. The more new cells you are making, the higher the chance that you can nourish them through effective skin care and diet to make them healthier than they previously were.

The hydroxy acids used for prematurely aging skin are glycolic (from sugar cane, which penetrates the deepest due to its small molecular size), lactic (milk derived), malic (from apples and pears), tartaric (from grapes), and citric (from oranges and lemons). The acid most commonly used for acneic and oily skin types is salicylic (derived from wintergreen).

When: Peels can be done every six weeks to boost cell production. They can be done weekly as an intensive treatment for aging and acneic skin until the issues begin to resolve, then lessening the treatments to every other week, then for maintenance and used in at-home products. If you buy peels to do at home, remember they will only be as high as 10% hydroxy acid and you can do them weekly as a deep exfoliation treatment. You can also use peels on your neck, décolleté, and the backs of your hands. Don't over use hydroxy's to the point of irritation, do use your SPF, and try to stay out of the sun to keep those new cells damage free!

Love Note: If you are using a medically prescribed exfoliant such as a retinol, a derivative of retinol, or hydroxy acids, you should only use an enzyme based exfoliant at home.

EXFOLIANT RECOMMENDATIONS BY SKIN TYPE

All Skin Types

Enzyme Peeling Cream $17, Pineapple Enzyme Scrub $16 www.RayaSpa.com Call to order.

So Refined (Jojoba and Mint Facial Scrub) $12.75 www.kissmyface.com

Rejuvenating Facial Peel (enzyme) $38.95 www.lbri.com

Combination Skin

Baborganic Crystal Face Scrub $34 www.Babor.com

Jojoba Microbead Purifying Polish $35 www.RenSkincare.com

SMART ESSENTIALS™ Daily Detox Scrub $6.79+
www.aveeno.com

Oily Skin

Almond Honey Scrub $15 www.RayaSpa.com

Cleansing Mild Peeling Scrub $24 www.Babor.com

Skin Prep Scrub $32 www.Dermalogica.com

Neutrogena® Naturals Purifying Pore Scrub $7.49
www.neutrogena.com

Exfoliate Foaming Cleanser $32.95
www.Sukiskincare.com

Acneic Skin

Enzyme Peeling Cream $17 www.RayaSpa.com

Glycol Lactic Radiance Renewal Mask $55
www.RenSkincare.com

Renewal Bio-Resurfacing Facial Peel $82.50
www.Sukiskincare.com

Sensitive / Reactive Skin

Enzyme Peeling Cream $17 www.RayaSpa.com

F10 Smooth and Renew Mask $37
www.RenSkincare.com

Olive Essence® Organic Face Scrub $24.99
www.HomeSpaCollection.com

Prematurely Aging Skin

Micro-Dermabrasion Cream $17 www.RayaSpa.com

Baborganic Biological Enzyme Cleanser $34
www.Babor.com

Hydra Mar® Face Scrub Anti-Aging $29.99
www.HomeSpaCollection.com

Dry / Mature Skin

Pumice Peel $51 www.bioelements.com

Pumpkin Enzyme Puree $16 www.RayaSpa.com

Nature's Solution Corrective Facial Scrub $19.99
www.HomeSpaCollection.com

Home Peels

Glycol Lactic Radiance Renewal Mask $55, Resurfacing AHA Concentrate $45 www.RenSkincare.com

Derma Cellular Skin Renewal AHA Peeling 10% $148
www.Babor.com

Glycolic Exfoliating Masque $15 www.RayaSpa.com

Gentle Cream Exfoliant $32 www.Dermalogica.com

Dermatouch Oxygen Deep Peel (enzyme) $36.99
www.HomeSpaCollection.com

Olive Essence® Organic Gold Facial Peel $29.99
www.HomeSpaCollection.com

Retinols

These are my favorites:

Dermatouch Oxygen Serum (all types) $25.99
www.HomeSpaCollection.com

Vitanol - A Retinol Serum $26 (normal, combination,
oily, and acneic, skin types) www.RayaSpa.com

Bio Retinoid Anti-Aging Concentrate $60 (normal,
prematurely aging, dry / mature, skin types)
www.Renskincare.com

Love Lesson #12

Serums

Serum? What's that? Serums are the most common missing link in most women's skin care regimens. Probably for these reasons: serums are more expensive and less common than other skin care products, and their purpose and use are not quite understood by the average consumer. I didn't know much about serums either, until I became a licensed aesthetician. It wasn't until I was studying skin care and using serums regularly that I began to understand their value. A serum is a highly concentrated product designed to deliver powerful, active ingredients deeper into the skin's cell layers. A well made serum will encapsulate the main ingredients in "vehicles" called liposomes and polymers. Think of the vehicles like a Mini Cooper, or any other "smart car," that will drive the ingredients quickly and effectively to where they need to go. Once the smart cars drive the products into the skin, they let them out to work their magic. If the Mini Coopers weren't part of the serum, the skin loving ingredients would essentially just sit on top of the skin and not do much of anything.

Serums usually come in liquid form or a consistency thinner than a moisturizer. This allows them to be easily absorbed by the skin. Serums are the product that can turn around the direction of your skin if it needs a U-turn. Hop in your Mini Cooper serum car and get moving! Serums have the greatest effect on your skin, whatever issue you are treating: lines, texture, firmness, discoloration, redness, acne, dryness—there are serums for all these cosmetic concerns.

How and When: For serums to work the best, they should be the CLOSEST product to your skin. These are the bras and panties of your skin care wardrobe. They are what set the foundation for everything else you are going to put on your face (and leave on). After cleansing, exfoliating, and toning—you apply your serum. If you are using an anti-aging or repair serum, be sure to apply it to your neck and upper chest area, also. I always remind my clients and students that your face extends further than your jaw line—it extends all the way to your breasts!

You should be using a serum both morning and evening. AM: I use an antioxidant for daytime protection, but you can also use one that is designed to inhibit oil and bacteria if you have acne prone skin. PM: Use a nourishing one before bed, since our skin is repairing while we sleep and utilizes what we put on our face to help. Acneic skin can use the same one as AM to keep from breaking out while asleep. If you live in a cold climate or have very dry skin, there are heavier, silkier serums with more viscosity to use on top of a moisturizer to assist the skin's natural barrier, the acid mantle, in protecting our skin from the harsh elements.

Eyes and Lips: Yes, you should follow the directions on cosmetic labels as to where and where not to apply products, however, many cosmetic companies recommend not applying it to the eye area, to avoid anyone getting it in their eyes, thus keeping the product away from this delicate place. There are times I disagree with this. When it comes to repairing and nourishing serums, I put them on my eyes and lips. Here's why: the tissue around your eyes and on your lips is delicate, it lacks oil glands and thus the ability to moisturize itself. For this reason, they begin to show the signs of aging more quickly than other areas. They need serums even more than other areas! The following Love Lesson featuring Howard Stern will help drive my point home...

SERUM RECOMMENDATIONS BY SKIN TYPE

All Skin Types

Vitamin-C Serum (the best) $25 www.RayaSpa.com

Serum 10 AOX+ (10% vitamin C) $86 www.SkinCeuticals.com

Beauty Booster® Serum $125 www.trishmcevoy.com

Keep Young and Beautiful SH2C Serum $65 www.RenSkinCare.com

Pure Power (red tea) $85 www.Goldfadensince1967.com

Vitamin C Serum $45 www.MarioBadescu.com

C the Change (Ester-C Serum) $17.85
www.kissmyface.com

Pure Uplift Face Firming Elixir $49
www.Oricolondon.com

Combination Skin

DDF Wrinkle Resist Plus Pore Minimizing Serum $85
www.ddfskincare.com

Hydrating B5 Gel $70 www.SkinCeuticals.com

Oily Skin

PHLORETIN CF $152 (vitamin C for oily and combi-
nation skins) www.Skinceuticals.com

Fruit Enzyme Serum $24 www.RayaSpa.com

Oil Absorber Face Treatment $35
www.lancerskincare.com

Acneic Skin

Blemish Control Gel $23, and Pro-Clear Treatment Gel
$24 www.RayaSpa.com

Resurfacing AHA Concentrate $45
www.RenSkincare.com

ClearCalm 3 Replenishing Night Serum $30
www.RenSkincare.com

Break Out (Botanical Acne Gel) $16.15
www.kissmyface.com

Sensitive Skin

Skin Refining Concentrate $26 www.RayaSpa.com

SkinLogics Sensitive Protective Services Calming Fluid
$28 www.BeautiControl.com

Phyto Corrective Gel $60 www.SkinCeuticals.com

Hydra-Calm Youth Defense Serum $60
www.RenSkincare.com

Prematurely Aging Skin

Vitanol-A Retinol Serum $26 www.RayaSpa.com

C E Ferulic (extreme protection and repair) $145
www.SkinCeuticals.com

Rapid Age Spot and Pigment Lightening Serum $60
www.Murad.com

Perfecting Skin Tone Serum XK $33.49
www.drlewinnbykinerase.com Walgreens and Walmart

Cellufirm Drops $25 www.MarioBadescu.com

Radiance Perfection Serum $55 www.RenSkincare.com

Maxifirm Skin Renewal Complex $37.95 www.lbri.com

Dry / Mature Skin

24 Karate Gold Serum $35 (luxurious), Instant Face Line Lift (2 part system) $21 (tightens and firms), Lifting Elixir (Botox™ in a bottle!) www.RayaSpa.com

Age Diffusing Serum $74 www.Murad.com

Full of Grace Solid Moisturizing Serum Bar $14.95 www.lush.com

Lift and Resculpt Serum XK www.drlewinnbykinerase.com Walgreens and Walmart

Rose O12 Serum $80, Omega 3 Night Repair Serum $60 www.RenSkincare.com

Plant Stem Cell Serum $48 www.naturopathica.com

Wrinkle Fillers

e.l.f. Wrinkle Refiner $3 www.eyeslipsandface.com

Instant Dermal Wrinkle Filler www.drlewinnbykinerase.com Walgreens and Walmart

Love Lesson #13

Eyes and Lips

Howard Stern, the Beauty Expert. Never thought you'd hear those words used together, did you? I remember a Howard Stern episode I watched many years ago (when his radio show was still allowed to be aired on television). He always had "hot" women on his show. His interviewing style, if you are not familiar with it, could be called chauvinistic, inappropriate, or off-colored. On this episode in particular, he had an attractive woman in the studio and was pressing her to answer some personally uncomfortable questions (that she, of course, knew were coming). She happened to be wearing sun glasses during the interview. Howard kept asking the woman how old she was. When she refused his line of questioning, he guessed her age, asserting that she must be older than she wants him to think because of the sunglasses she's wearing. I will always remember the next statement Howard made: he said, "You can always tell how old a woman is by looking at her eyes, because this is the first place that ages." She took off her glasses and her twenty-something year old face immediately looked forty-something. Howard gloated, and I felt bad for her.

Howard's assessment is nothing new. We all know that the skin around the eyes thins, and we develop crow's feet, dark circles, and puffiness here. Yes, Howard, we all know the eyes are the first to go. But they don't have to be. Here's what to do:

Put your products around your eyes and on your lips. These areas need help the most, and often do not get it, because the labels caution you, "Do not apply to eye or lip area." You can use serums, gels, and light weight moisturizers, but never use any acne treatment, drying or medicated creams, or anything chemical or abrasive on these areas. Apply the product under the eye, and on the brow bone, but never near the tear duct or mucous membranes.

Direction of application is crucial: Inward on the bottom, outward on the top. Use this direction when applying or removing anything to and from the eye area—cosmetics, makeup, et cetera. Under eyes: Move from the outside corners of the eye, inward towards the nose. Above the eyes: Move from inside by nose, outward towards the temples. This way you are always moving opposite the direction which lines forms and fluid settles. You will be going in a clockwise direction around your right eye, and a counter clockwise direction around your left eye.

Exfoliate the eye area. These cells need to be removed, too, just like the rest of your face. Do not use large particle scrubs like the old "apricot seed" scrubs. Instead, choose an enzyme exfoliant or very fine particle microdermabrasion scrub. Some hydroxy acid serums and creams can go somewhat near the eye area. It is only the problem areas of the eyes you need to treat, like the crow's feet at the corners, the hollow part under the eyes, and from the brow bone to the crease. Never apply a retinol product near the eyes; retinol travels and will migrate to all areas on its own. Never apply any product to the eyelid itself.

Sleep on your back, slightly elevated to assist the lymph drainage that accumulates overnight.

Cool as a Cucumber... Do cucumbers really reduce puffiness? Yes. Cucumbers contain the botanical cucumis sativis, as well as antioxidants and water. All can benefit the eye area by reducing inflammation, hydrating and, if used cold, relieving swelling. So yes, they are helpful; just make sure you wash the cucumber and chill it before use. Use thin slices so they conform to the contours of the eye area. Apply with your head elevated for 15-20 min.

Eye Massage

Our tear ducts' functions, which move fluid away from the eyes, slow down with age. Fluids remain and cause puffiness. Massaging the eye area stimulates the glands and helps to move the fluid out. **How:** When you have cleanser on your face (preferably in the shower), use your ring finger to circle around the eyes. Use the same movement as when applying products—**Bottom:** move from the outside, inward towards your nose. **Top:** from the inside of eye by your nose, outward towards the temples. So, you will be making circles around the eyes, clockwise on the right, counter clockwise on the left. After you've made about 5 circles, start making small circles with your ring fingers, while still tracing the larger circles around the eyes. It should feel like you are drawing flower petals or a cloud around your eyes.

Benefits of eye massage:

•Moves the fluid that builds up while we are sleeping towards the tear ducts and out of the eye area.When left there, that fluid stretches out the delicate skin.

•Stimulates circulation to these delicate tissues, which need more oxygen and nourishment from blood flow. It also strengthens the blood vessels that tend to be weaker in these areas, causing dark circles.

•Massage tones the many small muscles around the eye area that cause the formation of lines. It's like exercise for your eyes!

•Use gentle pressure to massage the eye area with care when cleansing your face or applying product and you will not only see an improvement, but ward off the aging process!

Love Your Lips

Finally, it's time to give some love back to Angelina, the goddess of lips we all wished we had! You can increase the plump in your pout naturally or, at the very least, keep your lips youthful longer if you:

Scrub your lips. The lips can handle being roughed up a bit, more than the eye area. Scrub your lips with your facial exfoliant, sugar mixed with honey, a warm damp washcloth, or you can use a clean, soft-bristle toothbrush. By removing the dead cells on the lips and increasing the surface blood flow, you will plump and soften the lips and continue to stimulate new collagen cells.

Apply leftover products to lips. After you apply a product to your face, put what's left on your hands, on your lips. Serums, moisturizers, eye creams, this is what the pros do when you go in for a facial. Just "tap" them onto the lips. Go just outside the line of the lips to avoid the formation of fine lines.

Don't "purse" your lips together, and don't use straws. This contributes to "smoker's lines" around the lips. Stretch your lips into the shape you would make like the vowel "E" to counteract this movement, and massage around the lips to avoid muscle contractions.

A Wink and a Kiss

Don't forget to treat the eyes and the lips. They need it the most. The skin around the eyes and on the lips is the thinnest of the entire body. They age up to 36% faster than other areas, so give them special care by protecting them. Just be sure to only use nourishing and repairing products, and be gentle. Then you will forever outsmart Howard Stern, the Beauty Expert!

PRODUCT RECOMMENDATIONS FOR EYES

Keep Young and Beautiful Anti-Aging Eye Cream $40, Active 7 Radiant Eye Gel $45 www.RenSkincare.com

HSR® lifting Extra-Firming Eye Cream $79 www.Babor.com

AOX+ Eye Gel $85 (reduces puffiness), Eye Cream (firms) $70, Eye Balm (mature skin) $81 www.skinceuticals.com

Midnight Recovery Eye $36, Rosa Artica Eye $46 www.Kiehls.com

Aveeno Smart Essentials Anti-Fatigue Eye Treatment, "Simple" brand Revitalizing Eye Roller $9.99-12.99, Drug-stores

Lift & Resculpt Anti-Wrinkle Eye Cream $27.99 www.drlewinnbykinerase.com Walgreens and Walmart

Beauty Booster® Eye Serum $95 www.trishmcevoy.com

Eye Witness (Eye Repair Creme) $16.15 www.KissMyFace.com

Skin Renew Anti-Dark Circle Roller $13.09 www.Garnier.com

Hi Rise Rejuvenating Eye Elixir $35 www.OricoLondon.com

Divine Eyes $74 www.usa.loccitane.com

Smooth n' Firm Eye Repair Gel $30.50 www.lbri.com

Intensive Eye Treatment $15.99 www.puristics.com

PRODUCT RECOMMENDATIONS FOR LIPS

Antioxidant Lip Repair (soothes and hydrates) $38 www.skinceuticals.com

Mint Julips (lip scrub) $9.95 www.lush.com

Lip Tints (8 shades) $7.25-9.95 www.lush.com

Lip Resculpt 3-D (plumps and protects) $16.49, EN-HANCEMENTS Lip Microdermabrasion $16 www.RodanandFields.com

Mayday Mayday Rescue Balm $40 www.RenSkincare.com

Neutrogena® Naturals Lip Balm $2.99 www.Neutrogena.com

Coola Liplux SPF 15 & 30 $12 www.coolasuncare.com

Love Lesson #14

Moisturize Me!

Many women are "moisture phobic" because it's hard to find a good—no, great—moisturizer, isn't it? They are either too greasy, feel heavy or leave a film on the skin, cause you to break out, or don't do much of anything (sounds like a bad relationship!). Then, there are those of us who use moisturizers on our face that are designed for our bodies, (often, the inexpensive lotions). I am praying to the skin care gods for you. Please, do not: 1. fail to use a moisturizer, and 2. use body lotions on your face.

Why is a moisturizer so important? Well, have you ever shampooed your hair and not used a conditioner? Your face needs the same consideration. Your skin is busy doing things day and night, good things and not-so-good ones. When it doesn't have a moisturizer, it does more of the bad things like producing more oil, overworking the blood vessels and capillaries, and taking water from your blood stream to hydrate your skin. It gets a bit hyperactive. When you apply moisturizer, the bad activities in your skin become more passive and the good ones kick in, like cell reproduction, recovery, and nourishment.

I recommend using a moisturizer during the day that soaks in, leaving no visible look or feel on the skin. It should absorb completely, no matter what skin type you have. This will keep the skin lifted and firm. If you apply a moisturizer that is too heavy for the day, your skin will be too soft and possibly loose. Save the richer, heavier creams for night time. They can sit on top of the skin and absorb while you sleep. I classify any moisturizer by its ability to absorb into the skin.

Types of Moisturizers

1. Ultra-light weight or gel

2. Light weight

3. Medium weight

4. Heavy

If you can identify your moisturizers into one of these four categories, it will help you to know which ones are right for your skin and when to use them. The categories differ by its ratio of water to oil, and the molecular size of the ingredients; water and oil molecules are able to "bind" themselves together with their "tails." Picture a Yin Yang symbol: it's similar to that connection. This ability is called hydrophilia: oil that loves water. The heavier a cream is, the more it becomes "hydrophobic: oil that does not love water." Keep this in mind as we discuss the different categories of moisturizers.

Ultra-Light Weight or Gel

Products in this category will soak into the skin almost immediately, leaving no visible trace on the skin, sometimes even leaving it feeling tight or visibly matte, in appearance. These moisturizers contain mostly water or a gel like Aloe Vera as their primary ingredient, and little to no oil. Many natural oils can be refined to such a small molecular size by cosmetic chemists that the water and gels help them absorb into the skin, where they can be useful. Ultra-lightweight and gel based moisturizers usually contain hydrating and oil absorbing or preventative ingredients.

This type of moisturizer is perfect for anyone who has very oily or acne prone skin, because you still need to apply something to your face so it doesn't become hyperactive, but you won't even know it's there. These are my choice during the hot and humid summer months when you don't want to put anything on your face! You can use an ultra-light or gel product as your day and night moisturizer if you have trouble using traditional ones.

Lightweight

These would be products with a cream- or gel-like consistency. They will also soak in within 30 seconds, leaving the skin feeling like nothing is on it, while still providing hydration and nourishment. They differ from the gel category as they do not leave the skin feeling dry, matte, or tight. Your skin will feel "normal." This is my preferred category for daytime. They may contain a small amount of hydrophilic (water loving) oils that absorb easily, and usually contain hydrating and firming or detoxifying ingredients. This category can be used by those of you with normal, combination, blemish-prone or sensitive skin. They also work well in the warm months.

Medium Weight

These products usually have a balanced water to oil ratio, and the oils in these products are very water/skin loving. The medium weight products will leave a slight presence on your face, 30 seconds after application. You will know they are there even though they absorb well. I guess we can give these the "dewy" description. If you have normal to dry skin, these are an ideal day cream. If you have normal to combination, these can be used as your night cream so you can get something done while you are sleeping. Medium weight products usual contain ingredients that soothe, protect, nourish and repair, so you are usually getting more into the anti-aging with these creams. They have a typical "cream" consistency and do not leave a shine, but rather a light residue on the skin. I like these for fall and spring seasons.

Heavy

These moisturizers are the ones that let you know they are there. They go on and remain on the surface. They may feel greasy or very rich in consistency. They are mostly oil with anti-aging, soothing, repairing, and protective ingredients suspended within them. They may contain natural waxes and binders to hold them together. Heavy weight moisturizers should only be used by individuals with dry, mature, damaged, or sensitive skin types. If used as a night cream, they should absorb into the skin by morning, but if used during the day will leave a visible shine on the face. Some women want this. I only use these during the very cold winter months, when the cold air and forced heat are wreaking havoc on our skin.

Expert Tip

You can turn a medium or heavy weight moisturizer into one category lighter by adding a few drops of water to it. Add the water to the moisturizer when it is in your hand. If you get a moisturizer on your face and you find it is a heavier weight than you prefer, you can also apply the water directly to your face then. This technique will also help the other active ingredients absorb into the skin better. This works because the hydrophilic, water loving tails of the oil molecules attach to the tails of the water molecules and help them penetrate into your skin. Try it!

Don't forget: Bring your moisturizer down onto your neck and chest. Remember, your face extends all the way to your breasts!

MOISTURIZER RECOMMENDATIONS BY SKIN TYPE

All Skin Types

Ultra-Light Seaweed Day Cream (cream/gel, my favorite!) $21 www.RayaSpa.com Call to order.

Aloe Vera and Herb Soothing Gel $16 (hydrates and soothes, can be applied alone or mixed with moisturizer) www.RayaSpa.com

STREETWISE Oxygenating DayCream $42 www.OricoLondon.com

Hydrating B5 Gel $70 www.skinceuticals.com

Wrinkle Repair Day and Night Cream www.drlewinnbykinerase.com Walgreens and Walmart

Vita-Mineral Day Cream $45, Frankincense Revitalising Night Cream $55 www.RenSkincare.com

hydro gel $20-50.00 www.Vasseurskincare.com

Moisture Infusion Oil-Free with Aloe $34 www.purminerals.com

Advanced Skin Rejuvenating Lotion, Night Recovery Cream, both $15.99 www.puristics.com

Luminos Hydrating Moisturizer $24.95 www.keys-soap.com

Combination Skin

Beyond Hydration (gel) $36 www.bioelements.com

Daily Moisture (lightweight) $60 www.skinceuticals.com

Balancing Weightless Moisturizer (controls oil + anti-aging) $66 www.BeingTrue.com

T-Zone Balancing Day Fluid $52 www.RenSkincare.com

Botanical Kinetics™ $33 www.Aveda.com

Olive Essence® Facial Day Moistuizer $19.99 www.HomeSpaCollection.com

Oily Skin

Vitamin B Day Cream (AM & PM—matte and oil absorbing) $21, www.RayaSpa.com

Baborganic Pure Mattifying Cream (lightweight) $78 www.Babor.com

Day 25 Cream $20-$50 www.Vasseurskincare.com

Aloe Vera Barbadensis Jelly $17.50 www.lbri.com

Acneic Skin

Vitamin B Day Cream (AM & PM—matte and oil absorbing) $21 www.RayaSpa.com

Oil Control Lotion $39 www.dermalogica.com

ClearCalm 3 Total Clarity Day Fluid $40
www.RenSkincare.com

Outer-Peace™ Acne Relief Lotion $40
www.Aveda.com

Sensitive / Reactive Skin

Azulen Day Cream (medium weight, AM & PM—heals!) $21, Revitalizing Cream with Live Yeast (medium weight, heals) $21 www.RayaSpa.com

All-Sensitive™ $33 www.Aveda.com

Hydrabalm (medium weight, protective barrier) $22 www.skinceuticals.com

Hydra-Calm Global Protection Day Cream $55 www.RenSkincare.com

Prematurely Aging Skin

Bio-Hydrating Cream (medium weight—firms), Revitalizing Cream with Live Yeast, Vitaplex-C Revitalizing Cream (multivitamin), Fading Cream, Fading Gel $21-25 www.RayaSpa.com

Skin Smoothing Cream $58 (medium weight, repairing) www.Dermalogica.com

Spa De Soleil® Instant Glow Anti-Aging $69.99 www.HomeSpaCollection.com

Tourmaline Charged Hydrating Creme $40 www.Aveda.com

Under Age (Ultra Hydrating Moisturizer) $17.85 www.kissmyface.com

Dry / Mature Skin

Collagen Day Cream, Collagen and Elastin Cream (night) $21, Placental (wheat) Cream, Bio-Effective Cream (rich, regenerative) $21-26 www.RayaSpa.com

Emollience $60 (intense moisture, medium weight) www.skinceuticals.com

Super Rich Repair (heavy) $78 www.Dermalogica.com

Lift & Resculpt Anti-Wrinkle Night Cream $33.49 www.drlewinnbykinerase.com Walgreen's and Walmart

Ultra Moisture Day Cream $55, Sirtuin Phytohormone Replenishing Cream $80 www.RenSkincare.com

Superico Vitamin Rich Face Oil $47 www.OricoLondon.com

Divine Cream $102 www.usa.loccitane.com

Love Lesson #15

Masques

Masques (or masks) have come a long way since the days of powdered mud mixed with water that left you with a red, irritated face. Facial masques typically come in three forms: cream, gel, and clay. They can be very effective in getting the job done when it comes to a specific skin care concern. Think of facial masques like you would the once-a-week deep conditioning masks for your hair that you use when your regular hair conditioner isn't enough and it needs some extra love. Masques can be used in your skin care regimen in the same way; once a week, or whenever your skin needs a more visible change.

Types to Use and When

Gel

These masques are mainly used to hydrate and soothe the skin. Think Aloe Vera gel on a sunburn. Gel masques are helpful if your face is showing fine lines on the surface, or is "thirsty" and needs a drink. These masques usually contain soothing ingredients that are beneficial to red, in-flamed, or sensitive skin. Gel masques can be used as often as you like. Go ahead and apply them close to the eyes and on the lips. Plump them up and hydrate them!

Cream

These masques are designed for dry, mature, or stressed out skin. They typically contain oils and richer ingredients. Blemish prone skin should avoid cream masques until you have gotten the pores cleaned out with a clay masque (see next). Cream masques are best when used once a week, or more often during winter months. Your skin will feel more supple and firm after using one. Expert tip: Keep your cream masque in the shower, apply it and leave it to set while your conditioner is on, or while you are shaving. The steam from the shower will lock the moisture in and make the masque more effective. Like gel masques, cream masques can also be used on the eyes and lips.

Clay

These have to be used with a bit more caution than the gel and cream varieties. Clay masques "pull." They draw whatever's in the skin out. That includes oil, toxins, and moisture. This is what you want if your face needs deep cleansing. The clay masque absorbs whatever's in the pores, like a sponge absorbs water. It doesn't discriminate. How to use: Spread clay masques onto your face and jaw line (not neck—unless you have acne there) with your fingertips. Do not use a brush. Spread a paper thin layer all over, keeping it away from your eyes and lips. Clay masques can dry and irritate these delicate tissues. You must spread the masque thin or it will not dry, and it must dry to pull the oil and toxins from your skin. Leave it on while you read a book or do something relaxing, until it has dried all over. If you see darker spots or "dots" on the masque that look like they haven't dried, this is the oil or debris it has drawn to the surface. Remove the clay masque with a warm damp washcloth. Use clay masques once a week if you have combination to oily skin. If you have oily to acne prone skin, you may need to use them twice a week. Use clay masques in the evening only. Clay masques can reach debris that cleansers, pore strips, and even extractions from a skin professional can't. Once you incorporate a clay masque into your skin regimen, your skin will produce less oil and you can use them twice a month for maintenance.

Never underestimate the power of a facial masque. It can get the job done when all else fails.

MASQUE RECOMMENDATIONS BY SKIN TYPE

All Skin Types

Cucumber Ice Sorbet Cooling Masque (gel) $16 www.RayaSpa.com Call to order.

Skin Hydrating Masque (gel) $38 www.Dermalogica.com

Hydrating B5 Masque (gel) $52 www.skinceuticals.com

Fresh Face Masks $6.95 (in store only) www.Lush.com

SKIN BRUNCH Kukui Rejuvenating Face Mask $42 www.OricoLondon.com

Facial Masque $28.50 www.lbri.com

Combination Skin

Seaweed Fortifying Masque $15 www.RayaSpa.com

Spa Warming Trend Green Tea Masque (cream) $26 www.BeautiControl.com

Oily Skin

Mint Masque (clay) $15, Volcanic Mud Masque $15 www.RayaSpa.com

Clear Improvement™ Active Charcoal Mask to Clear Pores $23 www.origins.com

Invisible Pores Detox Mask $34 www.RenSkincare.com

Pore Shrink (Deep Pore Cleansing Mask) $12.75 www.kissmyface.com

Acneic Skin

Mint, Bio-Sulfur, Bio-Drying, and Blemish Control Masques $15-18 www.RayaSpa.com

SkinLogics® Clear Purifying Scrub/Mask $20 www.BeautiControl.com

Sebum Clearing Masque $43 www.Dermalogica.com

ClearCalm 3 Anti-Acne Treatment Mask $45 www.RenSkincare.com

Sensitive / Reactive Skin

Azulen Soothing Masque (cream) $15, Cucumber Ice Sorbet Cooling Masque $16 www.RayaSpa.com

UltraCalming™ Relief $43 www.Dermalogica.com

Prematurely Aging Skin

MultiVitamin Power Recovery® $46 www.Dermalogica.com

Skin Recovery Masque $15 www.RayaSpa.com

Age-Diffusing Firming Mask $68 www.Murad.com

Balancing Antioxidant Mask $45 www.BeingTrue.com

Dry / Mature Skin

Collagen Treatment Masque $15, Natural Lecithin Mask (cream) $15 www.RayaSpa.com

Drink Up™ 10 Minute Mask to Quench Skin's Thirst $23 www.Origins.com

Ultra-Rich Creme Therapy $35 www.bioelements.com

Intense Hydration Treatment Mask $18 www.BurtsBees.com

Love Lesson #16

Proper Protection

If you're going to play, you'd better play it safe. We've already discussed the type of sun's rays in the Love Lesson: "Sun Worship," and the effect they have on your skin. Next, you need to understand how to be properly protected when having fun in the sun and during other sun exposure.

Types of SPF

There are two types: chemical and physical (natural). Chemical SPFs are any SPF that has ingredients listed with complicated names like: avobenzone, oxybenzone, dioxybenzone, octyl methoxycinnamate, homosalate, and such. There are only two main physical SPF ingredients: zinc oxide and titanium dioxide. The difference is that chemical SPFs absorb into the skin, allowing the sun's rays to penetrate into the skin, and then scatters them once they are in. Physical SPFs sit on top of the skin and reflect the sun's rays, so they bounce off of your skin.

Pros

Chemical: Offer longer protection; can remain effective over long periods; waterproof (since they are inside of the skin).

121

Physical: Natural mineral; non-chemical; good for the skin; doesn't cause burning or stinging; fragrance free.

Cons

Chemical: May be harmful to the skin causing free radicals; may cause burning or stinging on skin and eyes; may cause eyes to water; may have bothersome chemical scent.

Physical: Can wash/wear off, or have an opaque white color (think of a surfer's white nose). Many companies now refine the zinc and titanium particles so they appear less white on the skin than the earlier formulations.

Another difference between chemical and physical SPFs is that chemical SPFs don't begin to work until about 30 minutes after applied (they need time to travel into your skin). Physical/natural/mineral zinc and titanium SPFs work immediately once applied. You can't go wrong with physical SPFs unless you fail to reapply them after you have been swimming or sweating. Combining chemical and physical SPFs is very common for companies to do and very effective as it offers protection on both levels. Look at your SPF and makeup ingredients to see which type it contains. I prefer only physical for daily wear, and using the chemical/physical blends when I am outdoors for fun and sport. If I am on vacation in a climate closer to the Equator, I will use a high number chemical SPF like 50-80 SPF, then apply a physical one on top of that. I know it may sound complicated, but it's not. SPF is like clothing for your skin, one kind that goes inside of the skin, and one kind that sits on top. The numbers, in my opinion: once you go above 50, offer the same length of protection time, because it's doubtful you'd be in the sun for as long as the math would suggest you're protected for (i.e. 24+ hours of protection with a SPF 50 for a medium skinned individual). Besides sunscreen should be reapplied every two hours, anyway, to compensate for sweating et cetera. It is the type of protection that you need to be aware of, and when to apply it; and it is your personal choice whether you want to use chemical, physical, or both.

Expert Tip

Combine steps! I like to mix my SPF with my liquid foundation or moisturizer. Many women don't want to use an SPF because it is an added step in an already long list of products to apply to their face, and they don't like the heavy feel. I get it, I feel the same way. So we eliminate that extra layer, by combining two steps: choose either your moisturizer or foundation, and mix with an equal amount of SPF. It absorbs better than the two layers on top of each other. If you mix your SPF with your foundation, it becomes a tinted protector. I do this when I am going outdoors but don't want to apply full makeup; this way, I know I am getting the SPF and some coverage in one step. If you have a foundation that is too dark for your skin, mix a little physical sun block with it so that it lightens it up and protects. Play around with mixing any or all three of them to see what you like.

BB Creams

These follow the same idea as my "combining steps" listed in the previous paragraph, and are the newest rage in skin care and cosmetics. It makes sense. BB Creams ("Beauty Balm") also combine anti-aging ingredients like the skin loving antioxidants we adore, with a moisturizer, SPF, and tint all in one step. Be sure to look and see what type of SPF they are using: chemical, physical, or both. BB Creams are great, and I support using them. However, do not assume you can combine all these steps into one, and get the same benefits as if used separately. You still need to regularly do all the steps in your skin care routine, to see dramatic results. BB Creams are just convenient if you are in a hurry, and are a "juiced up," tinted, moisturizing SPF.

Application: Be sure to apply your SPF past the jawline, onto the delicate area of your neck and upper chest AND onto the area behind your ears. These are the areas many women miss when applying SPF and other products. These are the areas the doctors "snip and pull" when doing a facelift. Don't forget to apply here or they will sag over time! Apply to the back of the neck and hands, too.

It is easier than you think to commit to using proper protection 100% of the time. You will guarantee yourself a future of healthy, gorgeous skin. So do it—not just occasionally, but every time!

SPF RECOMMENDATIONS BY SKIN TYPE

All Skin Types

Clinique City Block Sheer Oil-Free SPF 25 (no chemical SPF) $21 www.Clinique.com

Physical UV Defense SPF 30 $34 www.SkinCeuticals.com

Cell Mate 15 (Facial Creme and Sunscreen) $17.85 www.kissmyface.com

Organic Wear™ 100% Natural Origin Tinted Moisturizer SPF 15 (4 shades) $11.95 www.PhysiciansFormula.com

ENHANCEMENTS Mineral Peptides SPF 20 Powder (Light, Medium, Bronze) $29 www.RodanandFields.com

Face SPF Unscented $36 www.coolasuncare.com

Brush On Block SPF 30 $30 www.BrushOnBlock.com

Natural Sunscreen Lotion with Aloe $28.95 www.lbri.com

SPF 15 Daily Moisturizing Lotion $15.99 www.puristics.com

Combination / Oily / Acneic / Sensitive Skin

Sheer Physical UV Defense SPF 50 $32 www.SkinCeuticals.com

Face SPF 30 Cucumber Matte Finish (mineral) $36 www.CoolaSuncare.com

Aveeno Natural Protection Lotion SPF 50 Available in stores.

Prematurely Aging / Dry / Mature Skin

Super City Block Oil-Free SPF 40 $21 www.Clinique.com

Sun Protective Cream SPF 30 $21 www.RayaSpa.com

Cell Block-C® New Cell Protection $30 (physical) www.BeautiControl.com

Wrinkle Repair Daily Lotion SPF 30 $27.99 www.drlewinnbykinerase.com Walgreens and Walmart

Sport

Sport UV Defense SPF 45 $38 www.SkinCeuticals.com

Sport SPF 35 Citrus Mimosa $36 www.coolasuncare.com

BB Cream Recommendations

Maybelline Dream Fresh BB Cream (5 shades, physical only) $7.44 www.maybelline.com

Physicians Formula 10 in 1 BB Cream, Powder, and Concealer $12.95-$15.95 www.PhysiciansFormula.com

Skin Renew Miracle Skin Perfector B.B. Cream
www.Garnier.com

BC Color Tinted Moisturizer (physical and chemical SPF) $22 www.BeautiControl.com

Face SPF 30 Unscented Matte Tint $36
www.Coolasuncare.com

Skin Perfection Gel $57.50 https://perfektbeauty.com

Thank you for investing the time to read these detailed explanations about each step in your skin care regimen. It is important to understand the "How To" behind each of them. This information will empower you each time you are caring for your skin.

Love Lesson #17

Makeup or

Breakup?

Makeup: can't live with it, or can't live without it. Women usually fall into one of these two groups. The division would be between women who wear a full face of makeup daily, and those who do not. Which one are you? Women who are accustomed to wearing a full face of makeup generally do not like going in public without it, and have a quick system they can do in five minutes or less to avoid it. These women's special occasion makeup can range from 30-60 minutes to apply. Women who rarely wear makeup, may take a few minutes to apply powder, eyes, cheeks, and lips, for a special occasion and couldn't imagine applying a full face on a daily basis.

Common reasons women give for not wearing makeup:

I don't know how to apply it.

It breaks out my face.

I can't find a shade that matches my skin tone.

Makeup is bad for your skin.

I want to be able to go without makeup.

Common reasons women give for wearing full face makeup:

I look "washed out" without it.

I have uneven skin tone, pigmentation, scarring, or breakouts that I need to conceal.

I enjoy applying and wearing it.

I like how it looks.

Here's the truth on makeup from a skin care standpoint to help you decide whether to makeup or breakup with your cosmetics:

Makeup is good for your skin during the day (while you're awake), and bad for your skin at night (while you're asleep). You already know that, right? The deeper reason is that makeup is another layer of protection between your face and the world (like another layer of clothing for your skin). The more distance you can put between what's out there and your skin, the better. The pigments in makeup are often made from natural minerals like mica, titanium, and zinc. Their opaque qualities help to keep the sun's rays, harsh elements, and pollution away from your skin.

I once consulted with a client in her late forties, who had the skin of someone in her early thirties. I was even more surprised when she told me she had been a professional water skier at a theme park in Florida for the early part of her adult life. I would have expected her to have a large amount of sun damage and aging concerns. Apparently, the theme park's management required her to wear a heavy waterproof makeup for the performances (I'm guessing it was a silicone or oil based product). Luckily, she wasn't prone to breakouts, and told me she continued to wear a similar foundation after she left her water skiing career. The heavy base served as both sun protection and a barrier between the elements and her skin, like clothes on her face. I am not necessarily recommending the silicone or oil based makeup, rather trying to drive home the point that makeup can be beneficial. If the ingredients in your makeup are good for the skin (it's a natural mineral based product) you can be confident that makeup, rather than breakup, is the direction you are headed in.

Healthy (Mineral) Makeup Brands

Youngblood

Revlon

e.l.f.

Mirabella

glō minerals

Luminess Air

"LOVE YOUR SKIN" MAKEUP APPLICATION FOR ALL WOMEN

Do you wish you had one "go-to" makeup routine that worked for any occasion and with any outfit? Now, you do! This is a "Neutral" makeup application, meaning it involves techniques and colors that are flattering to ALL SKIN AND EYE COLORS because they contain equal amounts of warm and cool tones. These are the most common and default choices and steps used by professional makeup artists. They are quick and easy to do.

1. **Base:** Apply your choice of either: liquid foundation, BB Cream, makeup primer, custom blended makeup + SPF, or makeup + moisturizer. Apply to face and neck with a downward patting motion. Use a makeup sponge or brush. Match the foundation shade to the color of the skin on your neck. This will extend and lengthen your facial lines. If you are using an airbrush foundation, skip to Step 4.

2. **Conceal:** Pat concealer into the corners and under eyes, corners of nose, and other areas as needed. Use a slightly lighter shade than your skin for general use, a pink concealer for light skin, yellow for dark circles, redness or uneven tones, and green for excessive red or ruddiness.

3. **Set:** Work a powder mineral foundation or light diffusing powder over entire face with a small circular motion.

The minerals set foundation, conceal, blur imperfections and further protect skin.

4. **Brows:** Brush your brows every day! Using a shaping brow comb brush them up, over, and down: Up from your nose, over to the arch, and down to your temple. This will train them to have the proper arch. Up, over, and down… Use a brow pencil or cream and fill in the brow shape with short feathery strokes. Then use a shadow brush to dust a slightly lighter powder shadow on top of them to fill and set the shape.

5. **Cheeks:** Apply a golden pink/peach shade blush to the apples of your cheeks. Remember, your cheeks are not flat, so make circles as you apply. Bring the brush up to your temples and circle above the brows for glowing lift.

6. **Eyes:** Apply a taupe (medium brownish grey) shadow from your lash line to just above crease and extend slightly out towards temple. This is a color that is universally flattering to all eye colors. You can add any darker color into the crease for more depth, and any lighter color to brow bone and corners of eye for highlight. I have an iridescent and matte taupe that I use as my base for day and night.

7. **Liner:** Work a black eyeliner into top lash line and sweep the line slightly upward towards the end of your brows to lift the eye. Blend the line with a brush or cotton swab. It is up to you whether you want to line your lower lashes. Using the taupe shadow with an angled brush, gives natural definition. Work the black liner into the lower lashes

and set with the taupe shadow for a more dramatic look. Use a pencil if you wish to blend, and a liquid liner for a more dramatic look.

8. **Lashes:** Black mascara is universally flattering to all eye colors. Work it from the base to the tips of your lashes, slightly wiggling the brush as you go. Brush inner lashes towards your nose and outer lashes towards your temples. A good mascara is beneficial as it contains rich oils and proteins. Cheap mascara contains waxes and preservatives that can dry lashes.

9. **Lips:** Match your lipstick and/or gloss to the color of the inside of your lip. Stick out your lip like a child pouting to see the area I am referring to. This is the most flattering shade for you. When in doubt, choose the same golden pink/peach shade we used on your cheeks. This is the look you see on most celebrities and is commonly used by professional makeup artists. Draw a soft line with a nude liner just slightly outside of lip line. Fill in with the lip color, gloss or both. This will give you a lovely, full, natural pout.

And that's it! If you apply this neutral full face with slight adjustments for day and night, your makeup will always look polished, classy, and beautiful. You won't have to wonder if it matches your eye, skin, hair, or outfit. It will flatter it all!

ADDITIONAL EXPERT SECRETS

Blend: I once attended a class from a professional makeup artist who formerly worked for Playboy. When one of the students asked her how they achieved that signature glowing, flawless "Playboy makeup" (assuming it wasn't air-brushing), she replied with one word: blending. Blend all makeup so there are no visible "lines of demarcation" which are edges of color. Blend color on cheeks, eyes, lips, and jaw lines. To do this, have several different size brushes you use for blending only; don't apply makeup with them. After you finish your makeup, go back over any area where you can see a visible definition between one area of color and another. Blur the line with your blending brush.

Contour: Contouring is becoming increasingly popular as women see how it is used on celebrities and models to enhance certain features and downplay others. The difference can be astounding. Here are two things you need to know before you start contouring at home: light colors draw attention to an area and make it appear larger, while dark shades distract the eye from them and make the area appear smaller. For example, if you had a longer chin, you would apply a slightly darker powder or shading cream over it to make its length less noticeable. If you had smaller, deep-set eyes, you would use a light shadow or highlighter to make them stand out. Use light to enhance and emphasize an area, dark to shade and deepen or detract from it.

You can shade or highlight with all your makeup, to start subtly. Just ask, "Do I want to highlight or shade this area?" Then apply your powders and creams to create illusion. Practice, and make sure you blend well. There are many video tutorials available online; try different techniques to see what works best for your face.

Color Placement: When applying color with a brush or applicator of any kind, remember to place the brush down on the area where you want the most color—the most concentrated/darkest area—first. Whether it's cheeks or eyes, the first place you set down your applicator should be where you want the most color. If it's a crease color, set the brush down on the outer edge of the eye first, then blend inward. For cheeks, set the brush down on the center of the apple of cheeks then blend out in each direction. Foundation should be applied from the center of the face where you need the most coverage, outward towards your hairline and jaw. Proper placement will give you the most precision to your application.

Emphasis:

If you want your eye makeup to stand out, as in a "smoky eye," wear the same neutral shade (golden pink/peach is ideal) on both your cheeks and lips. This will draw attention to your eyes, because they will not be competing with the other makeup. It looks very classy.

If you want your lips to be the focal point, or are wearing a bold lipstick color like red, fuchsia, or deep burgundy, wear the same neutral shade on cheeks and eyes. A bronzer is ideal. Your lips will pop and the cheeks and eyes will look fresh and modern.

Clean Out Your Makeup Stash: If you are like me, you have a collection of makeup (much of which you never use) that you bought and have kept because it either it was a trend or you would like to wear it…someday… Maybe you are also on the eternal hunt for the "perfect" lip gloss. If so, it's time to say, "Good-bye." Your makeup collection is like your closet: you only want to keep the pieces that fit and flatter you. Also, don't keep your makeup in a bag! Keep it in an organizer or divider of some sort, and only keep the ones that you know are working for you. If you have those ultra glittery or wild shades you are certain that you will wear someday in Las Vegas, keep an extra stash in your cupboard or drawer that you can pull out for special occasions. The rule of thumb on makeup's expiration is one year. Mascara should be thrown away every 3 months. (I know, I know, I have makeup from over five years ago, too.) Who doesn't need an excuse to buy more?

The goal of wearing makeup is to enhance your beautiful features and bring them out, rather than to camouflage them and create features that are not your own. Makeup can help the world see your gorgeous attributes, amplified.

It can give you a sense of confidence knowing that you are wearing makeup that complements you.

MAKEUP RECOMMENDATIONS FOR "LOVE YOUR SKIN" APPLICATION

Makeup Primers

e.l.f Mineral Eye Shadow Primer $3 www.eyeslipsface.com

Youngblood Mineral Primer $47 www.ybskin.com

Foundation

ColorStay Aqua™ Mineral Makeup $11.95 www.Revlon.com

e.l.f. Mineral Powder Foundation SPF15 $5 (13 shades) www.eyeslipsface.com

Youngblood Liquid Mineral Foundation $47 (9 shades) www.ybskin.com

glō minerals Pressed Base $43 (21 shades) www.gloprofessional.com

Smooth Minerals Pressed and Powder Foundation (12 shades) $11-12 www.Avon.com

Inner Light™ Dual Mineral Foundation (9 shades) $24 www.Aveda.com

4 in 1 Pressed Mineral Makeup SPF 15 (10 shades) $26
www.purminerals.com

Perfect Finish Liquid Foundation $18.50 www.lbri.com

Concealer

Advanced Concealer and All About Eyes Concealer
$16.50 www.clinique.com

e.l.f. Mineral Concealer $5 (5 shades)
www.eyeslipsface.com

Ultimate Mineral Concealer (5 shades) $30
www.ybskin.com

Powders

e.l.f. Photo Finish Mineral Booster Kit $5-8 Sheer/
Shimmer/Yellow Corrective www.eyeslipsface.com

Hi-Definition Hydrating Mineral Perfecting Powder
$40 www.ybskin.com

Redness Solutions Instant Relief Mineral Pressed Powder $34.50 www.clinique.com

ColorStay Aqua™ Mineral Finishing Powder $11.95
www.Revlon.com

Mineral Wear Talc-Free Airbrushing Powder SPF 30
$11.95 www.PhysiciansFormula.com

Cheeks

Youngblood Crushed Mineral Blush "Sherbet" $22
www.ybskin.com

Smooth Minerals Blush "Blushed or Radiance" $7.00
www.Avon.com

Petal Essence™ Face Accents in "Apricot Whisper" or
"Hibiscus" $24 www.Aveda.com

Mineral Wear Talc-Free Airbrushing Blush SPF 30
"Rose" $11.95 www.PhysiciansFormula.com

Organic wear™ 100% Natural Origin 2 in 1 Bronzer
and Blush (3 shades) $11.95 www.PhysiciansFormula.com

Pressed Mineral Blush "Polynesian Pink" $16
www.purminerals.com

Bronzers, Shading and Highlighters

e.l.f. Mineral Glow in "Bronzed" or "Shimmer" $8
www.eyeslipsface.com

Uruku Bronzer $24 www.Aveda.com

Tom Ford Shade and Illuminate Duo $75 (available at
fine department stores like):
www.NeimanMarcus.com and www.bergdorfgoodman.com

NYX Highlight and Contour Powder $9
www.nyxcosmetics.com

Mineral Wear Talc-Free Airbrushing Bronzer SPF 30 $11.95 www.PhysiciansFormula.com

Eyeshadow

e.l.f. Mineral Eyeshadow in "Socialite" (20 shades) $3 www.eyeslipsface.com

Youngblood Mineral Eyeshadow Quad in "Shanghai Nights" $43 www.ybskin.com

Mirabella Pressed Mineral Eye Colour in "Chenille" or "Sienna" and "Gilded" $10 www.mirabellabeauty.com

Loose Powder Mineral Eyeshadow $7.00 www.Avon.com

Petal Essence™ Eye Color Trio in "Gobi Sands" $26 www.Aveda.com

Eyeliner

e.l.f. Mineral Eyeliner $3 www.eyeslipsface.com

Youngblood Mineral Eye Liner Pencil in "Blackest Black" $15 www.ybskin.com

Blinc Liquid Eyeliner (tube technology) in "Black" $26 www.blincinc.com

Petal Essence™ Eye Definer in "Black Orchid" $16 www.Aveda.com

Mirabella Eye Definer in "Smoke" $19, Magic Marker Eyeliner in "Black" $22 www.mirabellabeauty.com

Mascara

L'oreal Double Extend® Beauty Tubes™ Mascara $9.99-10.95 "Blackest Black" www.lorealparisusa.com

Blinc Tubes Mascara "Black" $26 www.blincinc.com

e.l.f. Natural Mineral Volumizing Mascara "Jet Black" $5 www.eyeslipsface.com

Outrageous Lashes Mineral Lengthening Mascara "Blackout" $26 www.ybskin.com

Organic Wear® Mascara (variety of colors) $9.95 www.PhysicansFormula.com

Brows

Youngblood Mineral Brow Artiste $40 www.ybskin.com

e.l.f. Studio Eyebrow Treat and Tame $3 www.eyeslipsface.com

Lips

e.l.f. Mineral Lipstick in "Nicely Nude" $5 www.eyeslipsface.com

Youngblood Mineral Lip Gloss in "Devotion" or "Embellished" $23 www.ybskin.com

Youngblood Mineral Lip Liner in "Pout" $14 www.ybskin.com

Youngblood Mineral Lipstick in "Bliss" or "Sorbet" $19
www.ybskin.com

glō Minerals Super Star Gloss in "Rose Gold" $18
www.gloprofessional.com

Nourish-ment™ Rehydrating Lip Glaze in "Mango Juice" $18 www.Aveda.com

Lip Perfection Gel in "Sunset" $24
https://perfektbeauty.com

LEAVE

Just call me the teller of unpopular truths…

BareMinerals Foundation. I would have no bias against this foundation (which is one of, or THE, founding companies of the mineral makeup revolution), except for the fact that it can cause breakouts for acne prone individuals. I have seen it many times, and experienced it myself. I can even identify a "BareMinerals" breakout by sight. It usually develops between two to six months of use, and appears as multiple small bumps under the skin's surface. If you are using this brand and have a breakout you cannot clear up, it could be the culprit. Get rid of it, and any brushes you used to apply it. The product must build up within the pores and eventually create the reaction to it. It will take a little while for your skin to flush the product out, so switch to another mineral foundation recommended above and give your skin some time and TLC, and it will clear up.

MAC Foundation: Oh, the trouble it has caused. Women love this makeup brand for its high pigmentation and quality. It started as a professional stage line of makeup, and the foundations are very heavy for this reason. They may have excellent coverage capabilities, but acne prone girls beware: MAC foundation can trigger a breakout after only one application! I can spot a MAC breakout by sight, too. It usually appears as deep pustules, similar in sight to cystic acne, located on the cheeks and jawline with smaller bumps on the forehead and inner face.

I do not have any red flags about the rest of either company's products, like eye, cheek, and lip colors; they are all coveted in the makeup world. I recommend staying away from BareMinerals and MAC foundations until they reformulate for acne prone skin.

Frosted Eyeshadow: Have you ever developed red, itchy, even scaly eyelids after using a product on your eye area? Usually, it is the heavy "frosted" eye colors like white, pink, yellow, blue, and green that cause this (not shimmer, but frosted). The culprit ingredients can be: D&C red, yellow, methylchloroisothiazolinone, and methylisothiazolinone, to name a few. If you develop one of these reactions, you must identify what product you used, discard it, and refrain from wearing eyeshadow until it clears, which can be up to six weeks in some cases.

When in doubt, use 100% mineral, allergy free makeup that is good for your skin and doesn't contain all the mystery ingredients! There will always be those of us, and products, that are the exception to the rule. My recommendations, both good and bad, are intended to inform you, and guide you in the direction that is best for you.

Love Lesson #18

High- to Low- Maintenance Skin Types

Is your relationship with your skin a high or low maintenance one? Do you have a Diva on your hands? It is time to learn exactly how to handle your type, and what to do to meet its needs. Each of the following types' profiles will include: the correct AM and PM steps, types of products, treatments, in depth information, and special considerations. Please read all the skin type profiles, as yours may change, and you will know exactly what to do for it if it does. Some types need more attention than others, and that's okay. If you have a needy skin type, this information will help you go from high- to low-maintenance skin.

The best advice I can give you on how to maintain your skin is this: keep it up on a daily basis. Build your skin care product arsenal. Have various cleansers, toners, exfoliants, masques, serums, and moisturizers. Think of them as your tools, or even weapons. Get to know them, and the effect they have on your skin. Then evaluate your skin on a regular basis. Look at it and ask yourself, "How is it behaving today? Which of my products will best address that?" Then use the ones which will best treat your skin at that moment. This is the most influential way to keep your skin in a healthy state. Don't just keep using the same products every day. Direct your skin to do what you want it to do, not whatever it feels like!

Next, we will cover the different skin types in depth, from the lowest maintenance skin types up to the higher maintenance ones. Refer to the Love Lesson "Skin Care Rituals" to refresh any of the steps in a skin care regimen, and for the product recommendations. We will get to know your skin and its type, on a personal basis. Please read through all the skin types not just the section on your current state, since your skin type can change at any point in your life, or throughout the year. Understanding all types can also help you make educated recommendations for your friends and family members who may be having difficulty with their skin. You are now even closer to having the skin you love!

Love Lesson #19

Normal / Non-Reactive Skin

Vanilla skin, it's fairly easy to please...it takes what it gets with no complaining! Non-reactive skin is the lowest maintenance of all the skin types. It pretends to not need much loving. This is not true, as it needs more than it leads you to believe. If you have non-reactive / normal skin, you still want to follow a standard skin care regimen. The BIGGEST mistake women with "normal" skin can make is thinking that because they don't have any real concerns with it, they don't have to do anything to it. This is a huge no-no because at this very moment you may have great skin, but the cumulative effects of doing nothing for your face will show up one day. Then it could be too late to try to learn about your skin and how to care for it. You would have a lot on your plate trying to reverse the results of damage from the sun, pollutants, and decreasing cell function, than if you kept your skin healthy all along.

DAILY RITUALS FOR NON-REACTIVE / NORMAL SKIN

Cleanse AM & PM: Use a non-soap based gel, lotion, or cream.

Tone AM & PM: Mist or apply with a cotton pad.

Exfoliate AM: Use a gentle scrub or enzyme 1-2 times per week in the shower.

Serum AM: Apply multivitamin serum 2-3 times per week.

Moisturize AM: Use a lightweight SPF cream.

PM: Moisturize with a medium weight or all purpose cream.

Masque PM: Use twice per month, Gel or Cream based.

Special Considerations

Professional Treatments: Get a Facial with the seasons, four times per year, or when your skin feels like it needs a "pick-me-up." See your physician for routine check-ups.

Avoid: Harsh products designed for acne prone skin. Avoid heavy products for dry and mature skin. Stick to light to medium weight products. Avoid damaging healthy skin at all costs.

Special Considerations: Please, do not ignore non-reactive skin!

Love Lesson #20

Combination Skin

Does your skin have a split personality? Can't make up its mind? Combination skin likes to have its cake and eat it, too. Dry and oily at the same time, acneic and sensitive. Combination skin is the beginning of high-maintenance types. You need to give it an ultimatum to help move it in the right direction. To balance your finicky skin, you must trick the misbehaving areas into thinking they are getting what they want. (Beginning to sound like a relationship?)

Most often, the number one thing all areas need is hydration. Water will balance the dry, oily, and sensitive areas. Sound simple? It is simple. You will need to choose products that are lightweight but contain plenty of water and lightweight moisturizers like hylauronic acid and sodium PCA. Lighter oils like grape seed, sunflower, Aloe Vera oil, and coconut oil (to name a few) are okay for combination types because they absorb with the hydrating ingredients and satisfy all of your skin's personalities.

The goal with combination skin is to bring it into a "balanced state" of not too oily, not too dry, not too sensitive, et cetera. It's like training your hair to part in a certain direction. Make your skin do what you want it to do, not what it wants to. You will definitely have to pay attention to what type of day your face is primarily having. Then choose the products that will help balance it back to a "non-reactive," low-maintenance state. The more time it spends being "balanced," they more it will begin to behave that way. Make sense?

You will need to keep up on ALL the steps in your skin care regimen. With combination skin, if you miss a step, it's likely to get out of line again. When you keep combination skin balanced for long enough, you will have tricked it into behaving. It won't remember all of its indecisiveness.

DAILY RITUALS FOR COMBINATION SKIN

Cleanse AM: Choose a creamy, lotion-type cleanser that produces a light lather or foam. A gel may be too drying, whereas a cream is too rich and not cleansing enough.

PM: Do the "Double Cleanse" we detailed in the chapter "Skin Care Rituals." Use a lotion-based or foam cleanser again. I prefer non-soap based cleansers for most skin types. If your skin is feeling particularly oily, use a gel cleanser you keep on hand for a deeper clean.

Exfoliate AM: Alternate between a fine textured yet abrasive scrub like a microdermabrasion cream, and a non abrasive enzyme exfoliant every other day to keep skin cells actively multiplying and to prevent the top cell layer from building up.

Tone AM: ALWAYS use a toner on combination skin. This is the most balancing step, which you know is the goal for combination skin. Often this extra step can be what it takes to get it to behave. Choose a non-alcohol, hydrating toner. Mist in the morning—remember, you can buy a spray bottle and combine half toner, half distilled water.

PM: Always "wipe" tone with a cotton pad for PM. Use upward strokes, and pat around the eyes.

Serum AM: A serum with a fluid, water, or gel consistency will soak into combination skin, and help to treat it throughout the day. Vitamin C serum is an excellent all around choice. Serums made especially for combination skin will regulate oil while also hydrating.

PM: Use a lightweight anti-aging serum, like a hydrating, multivitamin, or retinol serum every other day. Have several on hand, and choose based on what improvement you think your skin needs.

Moisturize AM & PM: A lightweight gel- or cream-based moisturizer is perfect for combination skin. It hydrates and moisturizes, yet absorbs completely. When in doubt, make your own by combining a regular (medium weight) moisturizer with a natural Aloe gel. Be sure to use a natural Aloe, without all the blue and green dyes like the kind they sell for sunburns.

SPF: Mixing a physical or chemical SPF with either your moisturizer or makeup is a great alternative for combination skin if you feel multiple layers are too heavy for your skin.

Masque PM: Use a hydrating gel masque or a clay masque twice a week, depending on how the skin is behaving. You can also apply the clay masque to the oily areas, and the gel mask to the dry parts.

Special Considerations

Get a facial with the seasonal changes, or as needed. Do NOT tan your face. This will lead to dehydrated skin, with an over-production of oil. Isn't that what we are trying to correct?

Love Lesson #21

Oily Skin

Is your skin hyperactive? Too much oil production can be exasperating and feels like a problem you can never get under control, the cause being the two things that regulate your skin's oil production: your brain and your hormones. They are two things you are not able to reason with, so you need to use products containing ingredients that lessen oil production and absorb what it has already made. You may have to search a little harder for products with anti-oil ingredients, but you need to use them over the alternative ones that strip your skin of moisture, causing even more oil production. That was the old school approach to oily skin treatment—deep cleanse it, dry it out, and don't put anything on it.

The new school way of thinking for oily skin is to deep cleanse it without drying or stripping it, and to give it hydration and products that allow it to breathe, with oil absorbing and regulating ingredients. Water is very important for all skin types, but it is mandatory for oily skin if it's going to slow down the oil production. Oily skin needs to be "tricked" the most into thinking it doesn't need to produce more oil, and this can be done if you are diligent. Reread the chapter "Water, My Love" if necessary. Refer to the cleansing section in "Skin Care Rituals" for the Double Cleanse, which can be a game changing tactic for oily skin.

DAILY RITUALS FOR OILY SKIN

Cleanse AM: Use a gel- or oil-based cleanser. Resist the urge to wash your face throughout the day if you have excessive oil production. Instead, check your water intake, and use mineral makeup only, from your foundation, powder, and concealer, to your blush, shadow, bronzer, and lip gloss. The minerals will absorb oil, and help to stop oil production. They also allow skin to breathe. Often the ingredients in non-mineral makeup can trigger oil production. Blot your skin with tissue as needed. When you cleanse oily skin during the day, you upset its pH, it makes more oil, and the cycle begins again.

PM: Again, use the "Double Cleanse" method we keep talking about. Choose a gel or soufflé (whipped) cleanser that removes oil, but does not strip the skin. Soufflé type cleansers are thick in consistency, almost like a frosting, but when water is added to them they foam up very nicely. This allows them to contain a large amount of ingredients suspended within them, almost medicinal.

Oil cleansers are helpful to oily skin because the oil is attracted to oil and will pull it from your pores. You could use your oil based cleanser as your first cleanse, and follow with a non-soap gel cleanser for your second. You can make your own oil cleanser by following the recipe in the upcoming Love Lesson: "DIY Skin Care" or buy a one- or two-step oil cleanser like: Babor Hy Oil ™ and Phytocative. www.babor.com

Exfoliate AM: Oily skin can tend to be thicker in texture, and has a tendency to overproduce cells. You should exfoliate daily to counteract this. Definitely use a rotary brush, and another exfoliant with either the brush or separately.

Tone AM & PM: Don't skip your toner! Use a cotton pad and do a "pat" tone. You can pour or spray your toner into the palm of your hand and pat onto your face. The hydration will satisfy the skin and balance the pH, slowing oil production. Never use alcohol based toners on oily skin. Remember, toners balance the pH and hydrate, which can slow oil production. Use a hydrating, clarifying (non-alcohol), or hydroxy toner.

Serum PM: Adding a vitamin A based serum at night can accomplish a lot for oily skin. It is drying by nature, in the sense that it stunts the oil glands but does not decrease hydration. Remember, when you are using a vitamin A product, you MUST use an SPF daily. I would recommend starting with an over the counter or professional retinol before you get a prescription one from your doctor, as you can then see what strength you need. Less is more in the land of retinol.

Moisturize AM: Use an ultra-light gel-based or mattifying moisturizer. Look for ones with the oil reducing and absorbing ingredients. When in doubt, a basic, natural Aloe Vera gel can be used.

PM: Do not skip moisturizer before bed! You need to trick your skin while you sleep, too. Otherwise, the oil will build up in the pores and cause a breakout while you sleep. Has this ever happened to you? It's frustrating. Make sure you apply some type of light moisturizer at night.

SPF: Use only mineral (zinc oxide and titanium dioxide) based SPFs only. They are slightly "drying," balancing oil and calming, too.

Masque PM: Clay masques are mandatory for oily skin. You can use them up to four times a week, and should until your oil production lessens. You may have to experiment to see which one works best for you. If it irritates or reddens your skin, ditch it. Finish with a moisturizer.

Special Considerations

Pillows: Be sure to change your pillowcases regularly. Use 100% cotton pillowcases only, so your skin can breathe. Avoid heavy hair conditioners, hair sprays and serums, as they will migrate onto your face and coat your skin. Always wash your face after rinsing your conditioner, in the shower.

Facials: If you have oily skin and you are not having a regular facial, it's time to start. During the extraction portion of a professional facial, the aesthetician will work the sebum (oil) deep within the pores, to the surface. When oil remains in the pores for a period of time (around 2 weeks), it turns hard and yellow. When the top of that oil is exposed to air, it turns dark in color, hence the term "blackhead." When the oil is trapped under the skin, it is called "milia" or a whitehead. Often, the only thing that will remove these pore problems is professional extractions. All the pore strips in the world cannot remove the stubborn ones, or what's deep down in the pores. FYI: When oil is new it is clear. When the oil in the pores is being regularly removed, the oil production slows down.

I had a male client in his late thirties, who had excessively oily skin; he told me it ran in his family history. During his first facial, I spent a long period on extractions, as there was a lot to be removed that had built up in his pores (I'm not trying to gross you out, really!). When he returned two weeks later for another facial, I saw there was less oil in the cleansed pores. He came back for his third facial four weeks later, and there was very little to no oil remaining. He reported that with each facial and extractions, he was seeing less and less oil production, throughout the day. Following his third facial, I saw him with the season changes, or every few months for maintenance. He was happy that his skin was now "normal" in regard to oil production, and was able to maintain it at home with a proper skin care regimen.

Those of you with hyperactive skin: don't dismay. It is possible to slow your skin down and return it to a healthy, balanced state. Stay diligent.

Love Lesson #22

Acneic Skin

Acneic skin is the highest maintenance of all skin types. The Diva, the Dominatrix, to say the least! It will keep you under its control as long as you let it. It is time to take the control back into your own hands and win the battle against acne prone skin. Acneic skin differs from oily skin when: you are regularly experiencing breakouts. Breakouts that occur any time of the day, week, or month. Breakouts that are difficult to control, and you feel like you've tried everything, to no avail. It is the additional presence of one thing that causes oily skin to become acneic skin: bacteria. Bacteria is on all of our faces—good bacteria, bad bacteria, and some in between. For whatever unknown reason, probably genetics, acne prone skin has oil production like oily skin, but when you combine both the oil and bacteria within a pore you get a pimple, or a cyst in worse cases. Because of this, most people with acne tend to over-wash their face, which strips away the "acid mantle," a thin protective barrier between your skin and everything around it. This weakens your skin's immunity towards bacteria! Do not do this, because you will have more breakouts and a vicious, never ending cycle. Look for products that contain natural antibacterial properties (avoid Triclosan) and oil absorbing ones, as well.

Please review the oily skin section. You will follow the same regimen, along with the steps below.

DAILY RITUALS FOR ACNEIC SKIN

Cleanse AM & PM: Always double cleanse. First cleanse is light. Second cleanse is deeper—use your finger-tips to work the cleanser into your pores. Use a non-drying, non-stripping gel, cream or soufflé, and always cleanse acne prone skin morning and evening. Teens especially have a tendency to reject skin care regimens. Proper hygiene is crucial.

Word of caution: many dermatologists "recommend" cleansers like Neutrogena and Cetaphil for acneic skin. I adamantly disagree. The reason they recommend these brands is because these products are "safe" for acneic skin, because they are not doing anything. That's right: the pH of these cleansers is very similar to your skin's own pH. If you remember, a cleanser needs to be slightly more or less alkaline or acidic than your skin to cleanse it. If it isn't, it would be like washing dirty, greasy dishes with water alone: nothing would happen. But it would be safe to use, right? (In the case of oily skin, slightly more alkaline reduces oil production. Cream cleansers are alkaline.)

I believe this to be one of the biggest duping of consumers, when it comes to cleansers and the label "Dermatologist Recommended." Dermatologists specialize in medicine, not skin care. They will recommend products that do very little, so not interfere with their prescriptions. If I had a dollar for every client who walked through my doors over the past ten years with acne, and wrote on their client information form that they were using Neutrogena or Cetaphil, I could have enough money to buy one of those companies.

Please, do your skin a favor and don't just continue to use a product because it's labeled "Dermatologist Recommended," if it's not making a difference for your skin. Remember my saying, "If something works, it works, and you will see a marked improvement. If you don't—STOP using it!"

Tone AM & PM: Pat, do not wipe, toner onto acneic skin. You risk the spread of bacteria. Use a NON-ALCOHOL toner and spot treat active blemishes with an astringent. Choose a toner that has natural, antibacterial and oil reducing ingredients like mint, camphor, yeast (vitamin B), tea tree, and rosemary.

Exfoliate AM: You cannot use scrubs on skin with active breakouts ("active" meaning that they have not begun to dry up and heal). Scrubs can irritate blemished skin and spread the bacteria or infection to other pores. You must, however, keep the top skin cell layer from accumulating and trapping debris in the pores. An enzyme (gentle, fruit based) exfoliant will do the trick because it sits on top of the skin and works its way down. Use them in the shower 2-3 times per week. Use an at-home hydroxy acid peel or serum 1-2 times per week at night. Alternate with an at-home retinol serum, if you are not using one prescribed by your physician.

Side Note: Salicylic acid: I am not a big fan of salicylic acid. Many over-the-counter acne medications contain it, and don't generate the results wanted by those who are suffering with acne. I believe the skin can outsmart salicylic acid and it just becomes a source of dryness and irritation. I prefer a mild glycolic acid in a toner, cleanser, or gel serum of 5% for acneic skin. It dries up the blemishes and keeps the top cell layer down. It shouldn't be used every day, but rather when you notice your skin's texture thickening or you have a breakout forming.

Salicylic acid does dissolve oil based deposits in the skin, but it is a larger molecule and can ravage the skin while doing so, if used daily. Back off salicylic if you see irritation or if it doesn't seem to be doing the trick. Alternate your products. Tell your skin what you want it to do, not the other way around.

Serum AM & PM: A lightweight vitamin C serum is an ideal choice, as it will strengthen skin's immunity against bacteria and have a healing affect. Choose an oil and bacteria inhibiting serum for AM and PM, also. Alternate them, depending on your skin's behavior.

Moisturize AM & PM: Acneic skin needs an ultra light, ultra absorbing moisturizer for day and night. This will allow you to use a moisturizer without being "moisturephobic!" If acneic skin has an occlusive product on it, it will trap in oil and bacteria and you will quickly see a breakout. Have you ever tried a new moisturizer, and within hours you break out? It's frustrating, I know! Some products that do not absorb completely act like plastic wrap, covering your skin. It causes perspiration, oil production, and bacteria retention. To avoid this you want to make sure a new moisturizer soaks into your skin completely, and leaves it dry to the touch. If it doesn't, I wouldn't use it. You also need to avoid the main ingredient that causes these problems:

Avoid Mineral Oil: You may, or may not, have heard the woes of mineral oil before. Either way, it is important to stay aware of its presence in any of your products if you are acne prone. It goes by several different aliases, and you need to look out for them all: Paraffin Liquidium, Petroleum, Isoparaffin, and Petrolatum. People hear the name "Mineral Oil" and assume it must be natural, it comes from minerals! Don't let the different names fool you, they all come from the same source: black crude oil. Yes, the petrochemical we refine to make gasoline, motor oil, and kerosene. This nasty stuff has caused the world enough drama—keep it away from your face and your body.

It is "occlusive," meaning it acts as a barrier, keeping things from going in and coming out of your skin. The good stuff can't get in and the bad stuff can't come out. It has been considered a "Group 1 carcinogen" (cancer causing) in its less refined state, and a "Group 3 carcinogen" when refined for human use, which means it's not "suspected" to cause cancer. Whether it does or doesn't shouldn't matter much, since there are many natural oils that can be used as a substitute and truly benefit your skin.

You may be wondering why skin care companies are using it, then. For several reasons: 1. It's cheap. 2. It has an indefinite shelf life. And 3. No one is allergic to it. Baby oil is mineral oil in its lighter paraffin form. Vaseline is mineral oil as petroleum jelly. It is used in these popular products because it is more stable in its longevity than natural oils like almond or jojoba, which come from plant and nut sources and can break down over time, or be an allergen for those with tree or nut allergies. Mineral oil is an easy product for companies to use as a lubricant and barrier when the goal is to protect or trap moisture within the skin. They can assume that it won't irritate, go bad, or cost them much. If you have extremely sensitive, dry skin (like a baby's chafed bottom); mineral oil may be an option. If you have acne prone skin, it is not.

If you do not have a tree or nut allergy, look for natural oils in your skin care. Natural oils absorb into the skin, are friendly with water, slow the skin's own oil production, and inhibit bacteria. Keep an eye on all your products, and pitch them if they contain mineral oil or any of its aliases. Any oil that comes from a fruit, vegetable, nut, plant, or tree is a better choice.

Watch for mineral oil and its aliases in your makeup, too. It is used in all types of makeup from foundation, powder, concealer, blush, bronzer, eyeshadow, and especially lip gloss and liner, which can trigger clogged pores and breakouts around the lip line and mouth. When in doubt, use mineral makeup. It doesn't contain mineral oil! Funny, right?

SPF: Use only the natural, mineral based SPFs on acneic skin. The minerals can reduce oil production, inhibit bacteria, and calm irritation. Often the chemicals in other types of SPFs can aggravate acne. Use mineral powder foundation if you are SPF phobic, which has a SPF 15—enough for daily protection.

Masque PM: Sulfur based, clay based, and gel based masques should be alternated and used two times per week.

Remember: Get in the habit of noticing how your acne prone skin is behaving each day, and choose your products accordingly. Don't just keep using the same products every day. Keep directing your skin to do what you want it to do, not what it wants to!

Special Considerations

Facials: Find an aesthetician that specializes in acneic skin. You will not regret this! Aestheticians have a tool called "high frequency." It's a small glass wand filled with argon or neon gas (It looks like a tube from a neon sign). When applied to the face it has an anti-germicidal affect on the skin and dries active blemishes. It is also important to have your pores cleaned by the extraction method, as previously mentioned. Your aesthetician can keep an eye on your skin and help you find the right products.

Aestheticians, however, cannot treat cystic acne—the deep painful breakouts that occur below the surface of the skin. They occur when a follicle ruptures within the skin, and oil and dead cells seep into the surrounding areas, causing infection. Do not attempt to squeeze or pick cystic acne, it will only worsen it. You must see a dermatologist or physician for treatment.

Medications: Take great care when considering medications like Accutane, antibiotics, topical medicinal grade retinol, and birth control, to regulate acne. You should first see a naturopathic doctor to find out if you can balance any physiological issues which are contributing to the acne. I, myself, battled regular and cystic acne from age 13-31, until I was diagnosed with disease and dysfunction in my female reproductive system. I ended up having a full hysterectomy at age 31. It was not an easy decision, but necessary in my case. After the hysterectomy, my skin is a lot clearer. I did not expect this, but it was certainly a positive outcome since my acne had been triggered from a hormonal imbalance I suffered since puberty. If I had known, or had the chance to treat the imbalance sooner, I may have been able to ward off the severity of the condition.

At Home Treatments: Blue Light therapy (available from LED Facial treatment devices) reduces bacteria, heals skin, and reduces oil. It can also lessen the red marks left on the face post-breakout. You can find an acne "Blue Light LED Device" on Amazon.com from $40-$250 (Regardless of the price range, they all use the same basic technology.

As with any such purchase research your options before making your selection.). Another at-home device which uses oxidization to sanitize and strengthen skin, thus clearing blemishes, is TEI SPA's OxyDerm: At Home Ozone Tool for Clearly Skin, $125. www.TeiSpa.com

PROFESSIONAL EXTRACTIONS A.K.A. HOW TO POP A PIMPLE LIKE A PRO

Do you squeeze a pimple or not? If so, when and how should you do it? There are countless opinions on whether or not to squeeze a pimple. Here's my two cents, based on over 10 years of clinical experience: If there is something inside of a pimple, it needs to come out. Whether it's a hardened oil deposit like a blackhead, puss (infection), or a combination, it needs to get out of the pore. Whatever is causing the problem needs to be removed. The longer it stays in there, the more aggravation your skin endures, which means more white blood cells are sent to the area, which causes scarring. I'm sure I will take criticism for this, but I know that people are going to pop pimples, so here is the proper way to pop a pimple, or remove a black- / whitehead:

What you will need: hand sanitizer, paper towel, several pieces of tissue, several Qtips, alcohol or astringent, and hydrocortisone gel.

1. Start with clean hands—washed, and sanitized with hand sanitizer.

2, Lay all your items on the paper towel, so as not to touch any dirty surfaces.

3. Fold a tissue in half, and drape it over the index finger of your right hand. Then bring the ends together and twist them in towards your palm, and hold the ends tight with your other fingers. Do the same thing with the index finger of your left hand. Now you should have both of your index fingers wrapped in tissue.

4. Place your finger on either side of the pimple and press and roll inward, down, and up, towards the pimple. You are going underneath of the blemish to push what is in it, up from the bottom and out, like a volcano. I know that's not the image you want to associate with your skin, but you don't want to just squeeze inward and down, because that will force the congestion further into the pore. Bring it up from the bottom. (If the tissue/finger technique doesn't work, or sounds too complicated: try using two Qtips, and replicating the same movement.)

5. Move around all sides of the blemish, squeezing until everything is out. If there is any blood, continue until you see clear blood or clear fluid (no debris). Then you are done squeezing.

6. Three Strike Rule: If you are squeezing and nothing comes out after three tries, STOP! It is not ready and you will only worsen it. Try again later.

7. Next, apply an alcohol based astringent to the area (with a Qtip) to kill any bacteria.

8. Apply any brand of hydrocortisone gel (not cream, unless you can't find any gel) to the pimple only. This will reduce redness and swelling. You could also apply a blemish treatment gel at this point, instead. I don't care what you've read online, don't use toothpaste!

9. Any clay based masque can be applied over night to draw impurities from the pimple and dry it up. Dab on pimples only, not the surrounding skin.

10. Use a hydroxy based toner on the area until it begins to heal, then back off and use your normal products on the area, once healed.

If this sounds like too much work, I do apologize. If you struggle with acne, it's worth knowing the proper techniques to manage a breakout.

How to Cover a Breakout

1. If using liquid foundation, first apply foundation using a makeup sponge. Gently pat—do not rub—the foundation in. Then apply concealer with Qtips (do not use your fingers or a brush) to the blemish. Finally, press a mineral or translucent powder with a makeup sponge to set and hold.

2. If you are using a mineral powder foundation, apply the concealer first, then the makeup on top.

3. Choose a concealer color that matches your skin tone. If you go too light, it will draw more attention to the area.

Other Considerations and Recap

•Avoid indoor tanning, it creates a vicious cycle of increased oil production and dependency on UV light to fight bacteria. Try a few minutes of natural sunlight early in the morning or evening, or Blue Light therapy instead (Blue Light contains no UV rays).

•Avoid cell phones and hands on your face.

•Wash your makeup brushes with antibacterial soap and dry them in sunlight, once a week. Use disposable makeup sponges to apply foundation.

•Avoid dairy products as they have been known to trigger acne.

•Rinse conditioner before you wash your face.

•Avoid heavy hair products.

•Change your pillow case every few days.

•BREATHE! Bacteria cannot live in the presence of oxygen. The more that is in your bloodstream, the stronger your body and your skin's immune system is.

•Reduce stress and boost your immune system. Take a multivitamin and mineral supplement.

•See a naturopath for additional herbal supplements to clear skin. Murad Pure Skin Acne Clarifying Supplement, and Naturally Clear Oral Supplement are options. Always be aware of potential side effects of herbal supplements, and check with your physician.

•Vitamins and supplements for acne: A, C, D, B-complex, omega-3's, zinc.

GRADES OF ACNE, CAUSES, AND TREATMENT

Only dermatologists diagnose degrees of acne; but you can learn how to recognize and treat them. Keep in mind that the root cause of acne is a genetic predisposition. You could take two individuals—one who was prone to break-outs, and one who was not—expose their skin to the same factors, and their skin would respond based on its genetic biochemistry. It's not fair, but the more knowledge you have, the better chances you have of outsmarting acne.

Grade 1

Minor breakouts that come and go; a few blackheads and whiteheads, with some containing pus, and some that don't.

Potential Causes: Hormonal fluctuations. Onset of puberty and isolated stressful incidents (i.e. event, test, argument) can spike testosterone and androgen hormones that produce adrenaline, which spikes oil production—leading to a breakout. Pregnancy, or the dips and spikes in estrogen and progesterone, due to one's menstrual cycle can affect oil production. Touching or picking at the face and an inconsistent skin care regimen can also trigger breakouts.

Treatments: Maintain a complete AM and PM skin care regimen. Don't miss any steps: cleanse, exfoliate, tone, lightweight moisturizer or gel, and weekly masque. Spot treat with blemish gel (day) and use a clay masque (night). You can dab Visine onto blemishes several hours before an event to reduce redness. See an aesthetician to have debris removed from pores, as this will reduce the opportunity for a breakout.

Grade 2

Many blackheads and whiteheads, with more pus and bumps than Grade 1, especially on forehead and cheeks.

Potential Causes: Poor diet, dehydration, smoking, lack of exercise, continual hormonal imbalances, improper skin care regimen, dirty pillowcases, makeup brushes, bangs or hat on forehead. *Retention Hyperkeratosis: an overproduction of skin cells, with a lesser ability to shed cells.

Treatments: Eat a diet high in fresh fruits and vegetables. Reduce processed acidic foods like fast food, soda, dairy, and sweets. Drink more than half your body weight in ounces of water, daily. Don't smoke. Get at least 30 minutes of cardio vascular exercise per day. Exfoliate daily, using all the various types of exfoliating methods. Only allow clean items near your face. Maintain regimen recommended for acneic skin.

Grade 3

Main characteristic is presence of redness and inflammation. Many infected and non-infected blemishes. No cystic lesions, all superficial. Usually covers entire face.

Potential Causes: Food allergies, especially to gluten and dairy, and/or a highly acidic diet. Excessively drying or irritating skin care products. Lack of oxygen in the bloodstream, or weakened immune system. Improper hygiene such as lack of skin care regimen, or touching the entire face. *Cosmetic Dermatitis: Reaction to a product such as makeup, hair product, or moisturizer that is clogging pores or creating an allergic reaction.

Treatments (See Grade 2 Treatments): Try removing different foods from your diet, one at a time. Keep a journal to chart any changes you see. Add the food back, to see if it is triggering acne. Dairy, grains, and sugars are the best places to start. Do the same thing with all of your skin care and makeup products, starting with the most questionable ones first. Make sure you are taking a daily multivitamin and mineral supplement. You may want to visit a naturopathic doctor or nutritionist to help you identify possible triggers.

Grade 4

Cystic acne, mainly on jaw line and neck in females, and cheeks and jaws in males. Blackheads, whiteheads, pus, redness, and inflammation are all present.

Potential Causes: Extreme hormonal imbalances. Prolonged stress, anxiety, and aversion to a life circumstance can be factors, as well. *Polycystic Ovarian syndrome, estrogen dominance, and perimenopausal onset (near-menopause can occur in the twenties for some) are common causes in women. Males usually have higher than normal testosterone and androgen levels.

Treatments: Since cystic acne is a rupture of the follicle deep within the skin (dermis), it can only be treated by a physician. Do not attempt to remove debris from cysts—they will spread to other follicles. Do not massage, use scrubs or other manual exfoliants, or rub cystic acne. Trust me, it will only prolong the cyst and cause more scarring. What if you also have superficial black- and whiteheads present? Well, you must be very careful when treating multiple types of acne, and should see a dermatologist about the cystic acne first. Also see a doctor (gynecologist) or naturopath about possible hormone imbalances. Have your blood work done. You could use the LED Blue Light device previously recommended. It can heal, and reduce bacteria. Consider diet, hydration, and allergies to foods and cosmetics as mentioned for Grades 2 and 3.

*See your physician for more information on these conditions.

You may need healing on multiple levels. Stress can often play a larger role for those with cystic acne. Try to eliminate what is causing the stress; it may not be worth the havoc it is causing your physical and mental health. Practice relaxation, yoga, or meditation techniques; whatever is right for you, to find peace and calm. You may need to clear your life and your mind, to clear your skin. You deserve to have clear skin.

Love Lesson #23

Sensitive / Reactive Skin

The second highest maintenance skin type, next to acneic, is sensitive / reactive skin types. Instead of dealing with breakouts, you are regularly dealing with redness and irritation. Sensitive skin is the Drama Queen of skin types. It flares up without warning, or because it didn't like something you put on it. The key to treating sensitive / reactive (S/R) skin is to calm it down and strengthen it. Sensitive / reactive skin needs healing. It needs products that contain ingredients that will cool it, soothe, heal, and protect it.

The biggest issue for those of you who have S/R skin is the fear of trying new products. I know you have to be extremely selective and do not have the luxury to experiment with products like those with non-reactive skin. So you end up buying very bland products, focusing on what they don't have in them, like fragrances, dyes, detergents, et cetera. Okay, that's understandable, but these products also do not have any ingredients in them that can fix and heal your skin's sensitive tendencies.

I have dealt with clients whose skin ranged from mildly sensitive, to deeply red and purple in color, with patches of rosacea and irritated skin. I am confident that, by choosing products with healing and soothing properties that repair S/R skin, you can turn your delicate skin into strong skin.

DAILY RITUALS FOR SENSITIVE / REACTIVE SKIN

Cleanse AM & PM: Choose milky cleansers that soothe and calm. Some can be used with or without water, for those of you with water sensitivities.

Tone AM & PM: Use toners that soothe. Absolutely no alcohol allowed! Remember, toners balance pH. Sensitive skin has an unbalanced pH, and a toner can be very critical in its recovery!

Exfoliate AM: S/R skin needs exfoliating, too. Never use a scrub or brush. You need to keep down the circulation in areas that are prone to redness until they are stronger, so choose enzyme based exfoliants. These exfoliants remove cells without scrubbing. Use 1-2 times per week.

Masque: Use gel and cream only. Gel masques work wonders on S/R skin. It's like Aloe Vera on a sunburn. They hydrate, soothe, and heal. You can use a gel masque as often as you like, 2-3 times per week if necessary. Use it near your eyes and on your lips, too.

Moisturize: Many with sensitive / reactive skin avoid moisturizers in fear of allergic reactions, and some sensitive skins are also prone to breakouts. Often, the wrong moisturizer can make S/R skin look and feel "greasy," thus enhancing the redness; this outcome can lead to no moisturizer being used. Sensitive skin desperately needs the correct moisturizer to protect, hydrate, and correct the situation. Look for moisturizers that contain azulen, cucumber, vitamins C and B, yeast extracts, and calendula.

Makeup, SPFs and Protection: Primers and mineral makeup provide barriers between delicate skin and the environment. I know it is natural to not want to put things on sensitive skin. Instead, use more products that are designed for your skin type, not less. Dress your face like it's going to war, day and night. It needs as much protective armor as it can get.

The minerals and natural SPFs are healing, calming, and have opaque qualities that reduce redness.

Special Considerations

Water: I know I am stressing this for every skin type, but that's because it is so important. Skin can develop sensitivities just from being dehydrated. Red, irritated, hypersensitive skin is a common reaction to dehydration. Often, the increase in water consumption and the addition of a toner, alone, can greatly improve the skin.

Avoid: I will not say what many others say: "Avoid alcohol and spicy foods." I like alcohol and spicy foods, and you might, too—just consume them in moderation. I will however, say this: Cover your face if you are in a cold climate, and do not expose your face to extreme heat or cold. PROTECT IT. It's just not worth the damage it will cause if it's exposed.

Synthetic fragrances, colors, and preservatives are common allergens in skin care products. See the Love Lesson "Love, Like, or Leave It: Product Ingredients" for ingredients to avoid. When in doubt: Perform an Allergy Test by applying the product to a small area of your jaw-line or inside of your arm first. If you have a reaction within a 24 hour period, it should not be used.

At Home Treatments: LED, Infrared, and Photo Light therapy: these are multiple terms used for at-home, hand-held, completely safe devices used to repair the skin. You can easily buy one online (Amazon.com). There are many brands available, and the technology is similar no matter which brand you choose. I have a personal one for home use, and a professional one I use to treat clients. I have had the most significant success treating clients with excessive redness and rosacea. I recommend receiving a professional treatment once a week until the redness is under control, and then once a month or every six weeks after that for maintenance.

If you are using an at-home device, I suggest using it 40 minutes 3-5 times per week. The directions will say to use it less; however, you should increase the treatment frequency for sensitive skin to heal broken blood vessels and capillaries, and to strengthen the skin.

Professional Treatments: Intense Pulsed Light (IPL) lasers can be very effective treating couperose skin. Skin with an excessive amount of broken capillaries and blood vessels, and redness, often has hyper-circulation, and the laser coagulates the ends of the blood vessels which have broken at the skin's surface. I recommend having one (or a series) of these treatments before you begin at-home treatments. This will give you the best results. IPL laser treatments are offered at med-spas, and by dermatologists and plastic surgeons.

Love Lesson #24

Prematurely Aging / Damaged Skin

Has too much sun and fun taken its toll on your relationship with your skin? Is the past getting in the way of loving your skin? If so, do not throw in the towel and give up! You can drastically repair your skin if you are willing to put in a little time. Remember that it is a living organ and is very responsive to both good and bad influences. It took time for the skin damage to occur, it will take time to repair it. You must think long term when it comes to your face. Damage that occurred as a child and young adult will show up in your late twenties. Damage from your twenties shows up in your thirties and so on. It can even take 15-20 years to appear.

My goal is to get you loving your skin now, and continue loving it your entire life. To do that, you must come to terms with the fact that what you do now will appear at a later date. You must repair the damage that has already been done. This mindset is the only one you can have. Don't whine about having to buy the necessary products or putting the extra time in, either. You are responsible for your skin. You must respect and care for your skin before you can love it.

If you have signs of aging on your face like lines, loss of firmness and discoloration, don't look back. Look forward to loving your skin and looking younger than ever. Damaged skin needs stimulation, nourishment, and repairing treatments and products. It can be done if you commit to following a daily repair regimen.

In case you are not yet convinced, let me tell you about a little thing called a "Thymine dimer." A Thymine dimer is what has been called "a cell on the fence." It's a cell that has been damaged by exposure to UV light and now has the potential to become cancerous. It also has the potential to return to a healthy cell again. That's why it's considered "on the fence."

I learned about these little buggers while working with a top pharmaceutical skin care company, and more so after doing some of my own digging into other research that's been done. Thymine dimers are premutagenic lesions that alter the structure of DNA, meaning that they are the phase of a cell before it becomes a cancer (melanoma) cell. Our body's own attempt to repair them is actually what causes the damage. The Thymine dimer can be repaired by an enzyme via a process called photoreactivation. However, the necessary enzyme is an old one, present in many species of plants and animals, but unfortunately no longer present in humans. This is what is happening when you get a sunburn. The pain and peeling skin is a result of your body's attempt to repair the damage. The good news is that we can give our cells what they lack to help them repair the Thymine dimers, without causing damage.

This repair process is closely tied to the Free Radical Love Triangle we discussed in the beginning of the book. The same weapon, antioxidants (vitamin C in particular), that protects against free radicals, is what is used to repair the Thymine dimers. It is up to you to help the Thymine dimer decide which side of the fence it is going to. (Please refer to Love Lesson #2 and information on cell damage.) Remember, we are now thinking about our skin on a cellular level. With the right preparation, we can get those cells over to the healthy side of the fence again.

Before we get into the daily rituals for prematurely aging / damaged skin, let me preface it by saying this: You must use multiple types of products in each step of your regimen. It is like using multiple exercises in a new personal training program. Whether you are transforming your body or your skin, you need to change it up to make things happen. We need to hit your skin from every direction possible. Every product you put on prematurely aging skin should be doing something, actively making changes. Don't waste your opportunities by using "empty calorie" products—products with no repairing or protecting abilities. Let's get started!

Daily Rituals for Prematurely Aging / Damaged Skin

Cleanse AM & PM: Choose cleansers that have nourishing vitamins and/or exfoliating properties. Do facial massage in the shower. See Love Lesson # 31: "Expert Tips."

Tone AM & PM: Alternate between an exfoliating toner (hydroxy acid) and a nourishing, repairing, hydrating (antioxidant) one. Wipe tone with a cotton pad. You can dampen the pad before applying to dilute a strong toner.

Exfoliate AM: Cells that have been damaged also have diminished cell functions. Sluggish cells lead to lines, loss of firmness, elasticity, and hyper-pigmentation. You have to keep your cells stimulated by using multiple exfoliating products to encourage cell renewal.

Exfoliate every day in the shower. Change your exfoliant. Alternate between a scrub (like a microdermabrasion cream), an enzyme, and a hydroxy peel. Learn how each one affects your skin, and use a different one each time to keep cells on their toes.

Serum AM: Use a vitamin C or multivitamin serum every day, or every other day at minimum. Let it sit for several minutes before applying other products.

PM: Alternate between a topical vitamin A (retinol) serum, and a nourishing or firming one. Note: Fading gels or creams that are used to reprogram cells to produce normal pigmentation need to be used both morning and night for 6-8 weeks before you will see results (or according to product directions.)

Moisturize AM: Use a firming or vitamin based moisturizer. Your job during the day is to keep your skin protected, and use ingredients that neutralize damaging factors like sun, toxins, and pollutants.

PM: Your skin's job at night is to REPAIR itself. It needs the right products with repairing and regenerative components to do so. Remember to look for those beneficial active ingredients high on the list. Every night provides your skin with 8 hours of regeneration time. In one year alone, that's 2920 hours of repair! That's a lot of time to get things accomplished. If you are not using repairing serums and moisturizers while you sleep, you are missing the opportunity to turn back the clock. Use a richer moisturizer for PM, your skin can handle it then.

You should have 3-4 different moisturizers, and 3-4 different serums in your product arsenal to vary the repairing properties.

Eyes and Lips AM: Use a light, gel based product to tighten skin and reduce water and puffiness.

PM: Use eye cream lastly, on top of all other products. A light emollient eye cream works best at night. Pat from outside corners, inward.

SPF: While your skin is repairing, you must make sure it does not receive any additional damage. If it does, your skin will have to stop repairing itself to address the damage that is taking place. Lessen the damage, increase the repair. Load up on as much SPF as you can: in your day cream, as its own layer, in your regular makeup, or as your mineral makeup.

Masque: Use a repairing cream masque, full of vitamins and natural oils, twice a week: AM in the shower, or PM for 20 minutes.

Special Considerations:

Prematurely aging / damaged skin will need to seek treatment from a skin care professional more often than the other skin types. Once you have rejuvenated your skin, you will only need to visit specialists for maintenance. Please remember that damage didn't occur overnight, and it cannot be repaired in one day, either. Treatments that make drastic changes in one day alone are merely superficial, not addressing the cause but only the appearance. Receiving treatments that are repairing cells is what drastically turns back the hands of time, and gives your skin a more natural, rejuvenated appearance.

At Home: Use an Infrared LED device (available on Amazon.com) for 40 minutes, 3-5 times per week. Use daily in extreme cases. This increases circulation and nourishment, which encourages fibroblast activity in cells, which is exactly what you want to happen.

Microcurrent technology uses low level electrical impulses, similar to those produced by your body, to lift and firm facial muscles. TEI Spa's "The Tool" $140, is ideal for home use and they offer clinical trial results from their website. www.TeiSpa.com

Aesthetician: Receive a spa facial every 4-6 weeks. Choose: Seaweed, Vitamin, Hydroxy Peels, LED Photo Facials, Microcurrent, and Ultrasound treatments.

Nurse / Med Spa: If you choose to have Botox™, fillers, or microdermabrasion.

Dermatologist / Plastic Surgeon: High strength hydroxy peels, Thermage®, IPL lasers for hyper-pigmentation and broken blood vessels, Fraxel ™ skin tightening lasers.

I have tried everything listed above minus Botox™ and Thermage®. My skin was very damaged from sun exposure and other stressors. At age 27, I began to change my skin care regimen and what I exposed my skin to. I began trying all the treatments above, and using a full at-home product regimen. I am happy to say my skin is in better condition now than it was 10 years ago. Far better.

Your skin's health is more important than just its appearance. If your skin has been damaged, repairing it and protecting it improves your health, and lessens the risk for skin cancer and other conditions in the future. You are doing the right thing by making the choice to care for your skin. It goes well beyond cosmetic, in benefits.

Love Lesson #25

Mature / Dry Skin

Don't count mature skin out. It still has plenty of life left in it! Mature skin doesn't have to be considered "old" or "damaged" skin; it is generally postmenopausal skin that just needs special considerations. It can regain its youthful look again. Some women find that their skin looks and feels better during this phase of life than when their hormones were active.

You don't have to resign yourself to "looking old." Mature skin needs nourishment, repair, and protection, just like the regimen prescribed for prematurely aging skin. You can use richer products on mature / dry skin, since you shouldn't have too many concerns with breakouts. Choose products that are rich in natural oils like avocado, soy, olive, shea, coconut, wheat germ, and flaxseed. Select products that are mega packed with all the top nutrients like vitamins, minerals, proteins, amino acids, peptides, yeast, and other plant nutrients. They will act like super nutrition for your skin. You want to create an environment that will allow your skin to boost its cellular metabolism and reproduction, and lessen any aggravation and stress it may incur. Your skin may also fall into this category if you have always had dry skin, or have used a medication or undergone a procedure which has caused your skin to no longer produce any oil. Whether it is age related or externally caused, dry and mature skin types are handled in the same way: with care.

DAILY RITUALS FOR MATURE SKIN

Cleanse AM & PM: Choose a milky, cream- or oil-based cleanser. Make sure it is soap and detergent free, and full of lovely, rich ingredients.

Tone AM: Use a hydrating or softening toner with oils and water combined. The toners that require shaking in order to mix the ingredients are ideal for mature / dry skin.

PM: Use a stimulating toner at night that contains herbs like ginseng, gingko, or oxygen and alpha hydroxy acids.

Exfoliate AM: What type of exfoliant you use depends on whether your skin is delicate or not. If your skin is thin, use only enzyme based exfoliants. If not, you can alternate with a fine grain scrub like a microdermabrasion cream, or use the rotary brush in the shower.

PM: If your skin is rough textured, or you have very deep lines and discoloration, you will want to use an at-home peel product once a week. You can also use an alpha hydroxy serum or cream at night to keep the cells turning over.

Serum AM: Alternate between a vitamin C serum and a hydrating, plumping serum with hylauronic acid and sodium PCA, which are just like your skin's own natural moisture.

PM: Use an over the counter or prescription grade retinol serum or cream 2-3 times per week. Alternate with a heavy weight, high viscosity serum to soak deep into the skin's layers.

Moisture AM: Use a medium weight moisturizer with hydration and a built in SPF for daytime.

PM: Use a heavy weight moisturizer, the richest you can find. Add water to it; this will "wake up" the moisturizer by helping it deliver the nutrients to your skin. This is the only skin type that should be using heavy weight creams.

Eyes and Lips PM: Always put on last. Use a lightweight moisturizing eye cream. Keep away from corners of eyes as it can cause mature eyes to water. Avoid eye cream during the day for this reason. Apply to lips, also.

SPF: Use a high SPF of 30 and up. Apply on top of your moisturizer, as mature / dry skin can handle multiple layers. Avoid corners of the eyes, and use only the physical block (natural mineral titanium and zinc) since mature skin will burn, or eyes will water, when using chemical SPFs.

Masque AM & PM: Cream and gel masques can be used as often as you like, both in the shower and at night, to seal in moisture.

Special Considerations

At Home: Use the same Infrared LED device I have been recommending for the other skin types, 2-3 times per week, for 30 minutes. It will keep the cells healthy and re-pairing.

Microcurrent Device: This is something many are still unfamiliar with. It is a low current electrical impulse which stimulates muscles and tissues to tighten, lift, and firm them. It is similar to "exercise" for your skin. It is safe, and a similar, non-cosmetic treatment is often used by physical therapists to repair muscles. It creates a very slight "twitching" sensation in the muscle; other than that, there is no feeling. You can seek out a skin therapist or spa that offers microcurrent treatments, to see if you like the results. You can also buy an at-home device from Amazon.com. "NuFace" and "Serious Skincare" seem to be popular brands. Again, the price ranges from $40-$450. Dr. Lancer offers an at-home Microcurrent Power Boost for $225

www.LancerSkincare.com, and Nutra Face Lift Microcurrent retails for $195 www.NutraLuxe.net.

You do get what you pay for in quality, but as for the technology there isn't much of a difference (though the companies claim there is). I have used multiple machines. I own a professional as well as an at-home device, and both work well Spas use microcurrent machines that can cost upwards of 20K. These would be the Rolls Royce of machines. Like cars, they can all get you there; it's the quality of the ride that you're paying for.

If you buy an at-home microcurrent machine (which I do recommend), it requires the use of an ultrasound type gel. Aloe Vera gel, and/or plain water works well, too (mist water on dry skin or on top of gel). You must be open to learning how to use the device and taking the time to do it. Use it as directed—generally one to two times a week, and before an event. Studies have been done on the body (not the face) which show significant reduction in wound healing using low level electrical tissue stimulation when used for one hour each day. You can use it on your entire body, to lift and tone.

Professional Treatments: See the Love Lesson "Friends With Benefits." You can decide on whatever treatment you feel will help you love your skin!

I often hear women with mature skin say, "Oh, there is nothing I can do to change my skin. It's never going to look young again." Please do not adopt this attitude. The goal is not to try to make you look an age that you are not, or artificial. The goal is to give you healthy, radiant skin you can love at any age. If you take the time to care for your skin properly, you can—and will—love it.

Love Lesson #26

Body Conscious

Don't forget about your body—it needs love, too! So far, most of our discussion of skin care has been directed towards your face, neck, and décolleté. Many of these Love Lessons can also be applied to the body; however, the skin on your body differs from the skin on your chest, neck and face. Your body's skin is thicker and more resilient. On one hand, it can take a bit more aggressive treatment, but on the other hand—don't neglect it. The skin on the body is often overlooked when it comes to repair and protection. Your body should follow the same regimen as your face, minus a few steps.

Daily Body Ritual

1. Cleanse

2. Exfoliate

3. Nourish

4. Protect

Cleanse: Use a natural soap or body wash. Avoid using heavily fragranced body washes, and lotions that are perfumed. These synthetic fragrances are toxic. They offer instant gratification, and are very popular, but the long term side effects are not yet fully understood. Remember, your skin is an organ. What you put on it gets absorbed. Often, synthetic and chemical ingredients are more easily absorbed due to their complex makeup and small molecular size. You should only use natural, non-toxic cleansers on your body.

Exfoliate: "My body wash has exfoliating beads in it, isn't that enough?" This is another one of those 'if I had a dollar for every time I heard that' moments. The answer is "No." Beads in your body wash are not exfoliating enough! If they are not capable of removing the top layer of dead cells (like a texture similar to fine or medium sandpaper) then they aren't doing anything. My recommendation is to:

Dry Brush (see below)

Use homemade body scrubs (See recipe in "DIY Sin Care.")

Use exfoliating scrub gloves. (You can find them at most stores with the shower puffs and body brushes.) Use them with your shower gel or soap and really scrub your skin, paying attention to the areas prone to bumps, ingrown hairs, or dry skin like the bikini line, elbows, knees, inner thighs, back of arms, and butt. Scrub until your skin is lightly flushed with circulation. It needs the blood flow brought to the surface regularly in order to detoxify and nourish cells.

Moisturize: Choose body lotions that are rich in natural oils and nutrients. If you are using a drugstore brand lotion on your skin, 1. It may not be doing anything, 2. It may contain harmful ingredients like mineral oil and parabens, and 3. Your body deserves a better treatment.

You can also choose lotions that contain hydroxy acid to exfoliate, caffeine to stimulate, and algae to firm and detoxify. Your body's skin needs the nourishment and real moisture found in natural oils to stay healthy, supple, and pliant. Add a few drops of your favorite repairing serum to your body cream and shake. You can also mix several droppers of the DIY vitamin C Serum to your moisturizer. This is beneficial all year round to keep skin protected and repairing. I've recently decided to start using my facial anti-aging products on my breasts—these delicate tissues need love, too!

One of my favorite things to do is keep a natural oil in the shower, (like olive, coconut, castor, vitamin E oil, or a blend of any of them), and rub it into my skin before stepping out of the shower. Remember—natural oils are hydrophilic with their water loving tails. The water helps the oils soak in so you won't feel greasy.

Protect: You must protect your body from the sun and other elements. It is a living organ, treat it as such. Many diagnosed skin cancers occur in areas of the body exposed to the sun such as shoulders, back of hands, legs, and feet—areas we often expose to the sun, unprotected. Use an SPF of 15 or higher on all areas of the body, don't forget your ears, the back of your neck, hands, and feet. Wear SPF any time you are outdoors, not just sunbathing. I like the natural "physical" sunblocks made of zinc and titanium for the body, as well as the face. Avoid the sun during 10AM-4PM when the UV rays are highest. Dark skin tones need protection, too. The pigment in darker skin may give it more protection from harmful UV rays than lighter skin tones, but dark skin is also prone to discoloration and uneven pigmentation. All skin is susceptible to damage, so protect it! Please remember, your paler, healthy skin is more beautiful than your damaged, tanned skin. The same holds true for women with dark skin who use bleaching methods to lighten their skin. Reject any of society's ill-conceived notions of skin color and beauty. All of our natural skin tones are beautiful, just as they are. Embrace yours with confidence!

Dry Brush Detox Treatment

Dry brushing is an ancient technique that can be used to detoxify skin, move lymphatic fluids (your body's waste system), and exfoliate. Your lymphatic system is like your body's sewer, and it needs to be cleaned and moved along regularly. It resides closer to the surface of the body than the general circulatory system, and it responds to the movement and pressure of the dry brush. Your lymphatic system also brings nourishment to your skin and takes toxins away, so it's very important to keep the lymph moving. Only exercise, light massage, and dry brushing do the trick. Dry brushing is an inexpensive and easy therapy that will improve your health, skin, and weight!

How To

Go to any store that carries bath sponges, shower puffs, shower gloves, et cetera. Look for the long, wood handled, natural bristle brushes. They typically only cost between $3-5, and you can get them online, also. (You can even buy brushes with vegetable source bristles that are vegan friendly.)

1. Start on the LEFT side of your body, and brush from the tops of your feet to your chest (do not brush breasts) upward towards your heart. Include: shins, calves, inner and outer legs, buttocks, hips, abdomen, and low back. Cover each area with long brush strokes up to 7x.

2. Brush hips around and down towards the groin.

3. Brush from your finger tips up to your shoulders (front and back of arms) 7x.

4. Brush your neck, shoulders, and chest, downward towards your heart. Reach around and get as much of the back of your neck, shoulders, and upper back as possible (still brushing down) 7x.

5. Repeat on the RIGHT side.

6. When in doubt, brush towards your heart.

That's it!

Tips: Only dry brush in the morning, as it can be so stimulating to your system, it will keep you awake if you dry brush before bed.

Don't miss areas like underarms, inner thighs, and behind the ears; brush gently. Be sure to do both the front and back of body when on each side.

Pay attention to areas where you have stubborn fat deposits, water retention, or bloating. These can be areas of sluggish lymph and accumulated toxins that need to be moved and flushed out.

Use a light to medium amount of pressure, and brush until the skin becomes flushed with circulation.

Take a hot shower and drink a glass of water afterwards.

Dry brushing can be a very powerful detoxification. Therefore, if you have any medical condition/history, please consult your physician before beginning dry brush therapy.

I have heard of oncologists recommending daily dry brushing for those who are predisposed to cancer, or have an area they are keeping an eye on.

Weekly Cellulite Treatment: We can't have a Love Lesson for the body without mentioning the other C-word: cellulite. Unfortunately, it is an issue women have to deal with. I have read endless articles and tips on diets, creams and exercise to reduce cellulite, and they are all very helpful. I have my own expert secret that can be used in conjunction with them. I call it my Cellu-Detox Stone Bath. Please allow me to share how it came about, and then how to do-it-yourself.

True story: I once had a student take my aesthetic class who was also a licensed massage therapist. She was a very voluptuous, full figured woman, yet had little to no cellulite. One of the other students happened to ask her "How so?" and she shared her secret with us: Stone massage. Apparently the state she obtained her massage therapy license from required a six week curriculum for Hot Stone massage certification. During those six weeks, she and the other students could only do Hot Stone massage on each other. They were doing it about three times a week, much more than one would typically receive it in a spa setting—(perhaps once a year, or once in a lifetime, or never!) She noticed as the six weeks went by that her cellulite began to disappear. The other female students in the class were also noticing the same thing. After the class ended, and for many years later, she continued to use the stones on herself while bathing, and remained cellulite free.

Ironically, being a massage therapist myself, I reflected back on a prolonged period when I was using hot stones in my bathtub at home, to alleviate sore muscles from doing massage! I was also (at the time of hot stone usage) cellulite free. Several years later, I moved into a home where I was showering instead of taking baths, and I began to notice the cellulite on my stomach and legs returning.

199

Is this link scientifically proven? No. These results and techniques are based on experience (personally and professionally). I believe that the stones bring circulation, detoxify, move lymph, and break up stubborn fat deposits, all which are linked to cellulite in the health and beauty world. Cellulite consists of localized areas of fat, water and waste caused by imbalances in the body's systems. These semi-hard, gel-like masses that accumulate under the skin can only be removed by three things: exercise (muscle contractions), massage, and dry brush therapy. There are also treatments using hot and cold lasers, available from plastic surgeons. Some massage therapists offer cellulite treatments that use deep massage and suction cup like instruments to rid your body of cellulite, as well. Here's how you can beat the bumps yourself:

AT HOME CELLU-DETOX TREATMENT

1. Run a hot bath, add 1-2 cups Dead Sea salts, sea salt, or Epsom salts (Epsom salts, at least, can be found at your local drugstore, and all of them may be purchased online.)

2. Add 5-10 drops of essential oils. My favorites: Grapefruit, Eucalyptus, Peppermint, and Juniper. All are great for detoxifying and circulation.

3. Add stones to bath water. (You can buy anywhere from a few to a whole set of the black Basalt stones online, or use smooth, round, well-scrubbed river stones.)

www.MassageWarehouse.com

4. Get into bathtub when water is hot, but comfortable. Relax and soak for several minutes.

5. Massage: Apply a few drops of natural oil onto two stones (the oil you keep in the shower already). Starting at your feet, take one stone in each hand and massage your body one limb or area at a time. Use long, upward strokes, and keep movements directed towards the heart. Use a medium amount of pressure, massaging the stones deep into the muscles, not just superficially. Work the stones into any sore areas of your body. Knead the areas with the stones as if they were hands. Massage your feet, calves, along your shin bones, front and back of both thighs, your butt—especially where it connects to your legs. Massage your stomach, arms, shoulders, and lastly, your face. Trace the stones gently over your face using upward strokes. Really focus on areas of your body that have cellulite or stubborn fat deposits.

6. Be sure to get out of the bath while the water is still warm, and take a cool rinse in the shower. Drink several tall glasses of water after the bath to flush the toxins from your blood stream.

If you do this treatment at least once a week you should begin to notice results after a few sessions. You can do this bath up to 3 times per week. I mean, who doesn't love a hot bath? (If you can't, or don't like to, take a bath—you could just use the stones in the shower. However, it is the combination of the soaking with the massage that works so well.) Soaking and massage have been therapies used for centuries in Europe and Asia. Balneotherapy uses fresh water. Thalassotherapy uses salt water. This is more than just a "bubble bath" and can aid in overall health. Here's to a smoother, firmer, nontoxic body!

Funny story: I had a client who was originally from Europe, pre-World War II. She was from a small town that was well known for its spas and baths. She told me that soaking was such an important part of their health and culture that there were even outdoor baths in the middle of town. She was on a stroll one day, and decided to take a soak. So, she climbed into a bath and soaked for a while… in the nude. Apparently, when you finish your bath, someone comes out to "hose you off" with a cool shower. When it was time to be hosed down, out came her ex-boyfriend, whom she had recently broken up with. He had apparently just taken a job at the spa. So there she was, being sprayed by her ex, in the middle of town. She said she couldn't have cared less, she was so relaxed from her bath. She always found it odd that we didn't have public baths in America. I'm beginning to, also.

BODY CONSCIOUS PRODUCT RECOMMENDATIONS

Body Washes $22-27 www.RenSkincare.com

Body Contouring Anti-Cellulite Gel $48, Neroli and Grapefruit Body Cream $29 www.RenSkincare.com

Love Your Skin: Expert Skin Care Secrets Exposed

Body Nourishing Seaweed Oil $19, Body Nourishing Cream $15 www.RayaSpa.com Call to order.

Lush Massage Bars (Moisturizing Solids) "Hottie" and "Mange Too" $7.95-13.95 www.lush.com

Shower Body Butter Bar (lotion and exfoliation in 1) "Buffy" $11.95-22.95 www.lush.com

Kiehl's Creme de Corps Soy Milk and Honey Whipped Body Butter $38-$48 (Oprah's favorite!) www.kiehls.com

Moisture + Repair Anti-Aging Body Cream $39 www.BeingTrue.com

ESSENTIALS Sunless Tanning Foam & Daily Body Moisturizer $24 www.RodanandFields.com

Body Jelly $12 www.CarolsDaughter.com

COOLA Hand & Body Lotion Bars $12-22 www.coolasuncare.com

Guerande Salt Exfoliating Body Balm $37 www.RenSkincare.com

Olive Oil Moisturizers (face and body) $11.95 www.kissmyface.com

Blissful Shea Body Butter, Organic Spa Lotion, Shower Gels $10 and up. www.soycandlesandorganicbathcare.com

Full Cup Bust and Neck Enhancing Elixir $47, U Turn Stretch Mark Elixir $42 www.Oricolondon.com

Body Perfection Gel/Tan $48 https://perfektbeauty.com

Body Butters, Scrubs, Soaps & Oils $18 & up
www.LaLicious.com

Leave

Talc / Talcum Powder: Please do not apply talcum powder (baby powder, fragranced powders) to your skin. Talc can be highly toxic since it is similar to asbestos in its chemical composition. It can be an irritant when inhaled, and potentially cancer causing if it makes its way into our organs. A quote by Ruth Winter M.S., "In a study done at The Boston Brigham and Women's Hospital, of 215 women with ovarian cancer, 32 had used talcum powder on their genitals and sanitary napkins." She goes on to explain that the study revealed that a woman's chance of developing ovarian cancer was 3.28 times greater when using talc.

I have two experiences with talc. First, when I was in my early twenties, I lived in a small mining town in New Mexico. One of the chief substances excavated from the mine was magnesium silicate: talc. I heard that numerous mine workers had developed cancer, or respiratory illnesses believed to be a result of the prolonged talc exposure.

Second, when I had just become an aesthetician, it was common practice to use baby powder as a buffer before body waxing. I had a large hair removal clientele, so I used quite a bit of talcum powder, and I began to develop severe allergies (that I have to this day). I started looking at everything I was exposed to, and was shocked when I realized that baby/talcum powder was actually talc. Duh. I now only use talc free, corn starch based powders on myself and my clients.

There are alternatives to talcum powder that you can buy or make. You could use plain cornstarch alone, to absorb moisture or act as a barrier. Add a few drops of essential oils like lavender or rose for fragrance. I have seen recipes that add several tablespoons of Arrowroot powder, rice powder, French clay, or finely ground oats, per ½ cup of cornstarch. Feel free to experiment based on what you have available.

Available online:

Gentle Care Butt Dust Talc Free Baby Powder $7

www.vitasprings.com

Burt's Bees Baby Bee Dusting Powder $6

www.BurtsBees.com

Love Lesson #27

Going Au Naturel

Prefer to go au naturel? Au naturel is French for "natural" or "naked," and you can't get any more naked in your skin care regimen than essential oils. They are the purest you can get. Essential oils and their benefits deserve some love regarding skin care, your health and wellbeing. They are extracted from plant sources like flowers, leaves, wood, bark, roots, seeds, or peels, by the means of steam distillation, expression, or solvent extraction.

Essential oils are one of the few things that can enter your system and then go directly into your blood stream—through your skin, inhalation, or ingestion—making them very powerful, and some of the world's oldest forms of skin care and medicine. Because of this, they must be used with care if you are pregnant, nursing, have any food, nut, or plant, allergies, or health conditions that may contraindicate the use of essential oils. Please consult a physician or aromatherapist. I do not specialize in essential oils exclusively, but I have used them personally and professionally for skin care treatments throughout my entire career.

If you are interested in learning more about essential oils, I have listed my recommendations in the Resources section. There is an abundance of information online as well. Keep in mind: you want to use only pure, therapeutic, grade oils. Some of the top lines available are Aura Cacia, Aromatics International, Young Living, and doTerra. The last two listed are multi level marketing companies which offer you the incentive to join their organization or to buy the oils from a sales member. (I am not personally affiliated with any company.)

Therapeutic grade oils can be inhaled, applied topically (with or without a carrier oil), or ingested (only a few).

ESSENTIAL OIL USAGE FOR SKIN CARE

•You can blend 1-6 drops (per ounce) into an existing skin care product (start low and work your way up).

•Custom blend your own skin oil by choosing a carrier oil and one or multiple essential oils. Add 15 drops of essential oil per ounce of carrier oil.

•Make a natural carrier blend by combining equal parts pure Aloe Vera gel, vegetable glycerin, and a carrier oil, with 5-6 drops essential oils per ounce of carrier.

•Apply essential oils directly to skin, with or without a few drops of a carrier oil.

OILS BY SKIN TYPE

All Skin Types

Essential Oils: Lavender: balancing and normalizing. Eucalyptus: revitalizing. Chamomile: calming and soothing. Calendula and Rosemary: healing. Cedarwood: toning. Tea Tree: all around antiseptic.

Carrier Oils: Jojoba, Safflower, Olive, Sunflower, Sesame, Soy, Peanut. Castor Oil: detoxifying (blend with other carrier oil).

Combination Skin

Essential Oils: Sandalwood, Jasmine, Rosemary, Pomegranate, Sage, and Calendula: purifying. Lavender: balancing. Apple: balances pH. Juniper: tones and cleanses.

Carrier Oils: Sesame, Grape Seed, Apricot Kernel.

Oily Skin

Essential Oils: Lemon, Spearmint, and Peppermint: to tone and tighten pores. Eucalyptus: cools and refreshes. Comfrey: reduces oil secretions. Fennel: cleansing and detoxifying (never use on children due to high potency). Lavender, and Ylang-Ylang: treat excessive oiliness.

Carrier Oils: Grape Seed: very lightweight. Apricot Kernel, Sesame.

Acneic Skin

Essential Oils: Peppermint: inhibits bacteria and reduces inflammation. Comfrey: reduces oil secretions, and acts as an astringent. Wintergreen: contains salicylic acid, antiseptic. Tea Tree: antimicrobial. Bergamot: skin clearing (do not use before sun exposure). Eucalyptus, Cypress and Lemon: antiseptic. Sage: purifying. Lavender and Rosemary: treat acne. Spearmint: decongests and clears acne.

Carrier Oils: Grape Seed: very lightweight. Apricot Kernel.

Sensitive Skin

Essential Oils: Comfrey: promotes healing. Chamomile: healing. Aloe Vera: soothing and healing. Arnica, Calendula, Rose and Neroli: anti-inflammatory. Sandalwood and Cypress: treat broken capillaries. Everlasting: very healing to all skin irritations. Rosemary: treats eczema.

Carrier Oils: Avocado: extremely calming and safe for those with allergies. Evening Primrose Oil: treats eczema, soothes and heals inflammation. Safflower Oil.

Prematurely Aging Skin (see Mature Skin)

Essential Oils: Sage, Lavender, and Rose: regenerate skin cells. Frankincense: stimulates collagen production. Ginseng: stimulates and oxygenates. Lemon, Orange, and Mandarin: lighten pigmented spots. Neroli and Patchouli: have rejuvenating effects. Benzoin Resinoid: rejuvenates and tightens skin.

Carrier Oils: Carrot Oil: repairs sagging, wrinkled, damaged skin. Olive Oil, Vitamin E Oil Capsules.

Mature / Dry Skin (see Aging Skin)

Essential Oils: Eucalyptus: stimulating. Aloe Vera: soothing. Frankincense, Sandalwood, Fennel, and Myrrh: firming. Rose: promotes cell regeneration. Ginseng: stimulates metabolism. Bay and Ginger: stimulating. Cinnamon: stimulating (always use with carrier oil, never directly on skin).

Carrier Oils: Olive Oil: softening and nourishing. Avocado: thick and contains A & E; both natural preservatives. Argan Oil: replenishes collagen and elastin stores, contains vitamin E. Almond Oil and Wheat Germ: nourishing and moisturizing. Peach or Apricot Kernel: emollient and nourishing. Vitamin E oil (you can open a capsule and apply directly to skin). Cocoa and Shea Butters.

This list is a place for you to start, for incorporating essential oils into your skin care regimen. They have been used for centuries and are commonly found in many skin care and cosmetic formulations. It is up to you to experiment with different oils to find which ones work best for your skin type, and discover the benefits of going au naturel.

Love Lesson #28

Do-It-Yourself Skin Care

DIY is all the rage nowadays. There are plenty of full length skin care books, websites, and blogs available on how to make your own at-home cosmetics (I've listed several in the Resources section.). I use some homemade skin care creations, but not an extensive amount since there are many well established cosmetic companies who spend millions of dollars annually on product testing and development. These advances being made in the skin care industry are ones to be taken advantage of.

DIY skin care is simple, natural, effective, fun, and a bit messy! It's inexpensive, too. However, you must remember that DIY recipes are not stabilized like traditional cosmetics, and some recipes must be kept in the refrigerator and are intended for several uses only, as they will expire—like foods. You can use them every day so they won't go to waste. You will need to shake or mix your homemade products before each use since they may separate. Also, DIY skin care is not an exact science, and measurements may vary.

I believe that balance in all areas of life is the healthiest approach, so I recognize that cosmeceuticals, cosmetics, at-home preparations, and natural cosmetics all have their place, and can be used together to benefit your skin in a well rounded way. They all have something to offer your skin; take advantage of them. Do-It-Yourself recipes are a great idea for a "Girls Night In, Love Your Skin" party! Here are a few of my favorite DIY recipes that I've gathered over the years:

Love Note: Unless you have an established skin care company, I would not recommend selling your homemade products. If someone has an allergic reaction to something you've made, you are legally responsible and considered "at fault."

A few things you will need to have on hand:

1. A good blender or food processor. I use a Ninja® blender to grind the ingredients for both my skin care and smoothie recipes.

2. Containers. Save your empty cosmetic jars and bottles (especially toner bottles with pumps—the store-bought kind do not mist finely enough). Put them through the dishwasher when empty, and reuse them for your DIY recipes. You can reuse empty food jars with lids, like honey, peanut butter, jam, et cetera, if you put them through the dishwasher, too. Use plastic jars if you will be taking the product into the shower. Tupperware storage containers

work well for larger batches. (When using high amounts of essential oils or storing long term, use glass containers, as the oils can deteriorate plastic.)

3. Small glass bowl or ramekins for mixing.

4. Small funnel (available in baking section or hardware store).

5. Vitamin A and E capsules, and vitamin C powder. You can add anywhere from a few drops to the entire A/E capsule to your recipes, as natural preservatives, or a pinch of your vitamin C powder.

6. Most of the oils, bases, and bottles can be bought at your local health food store or at Amazon.com

LYS Vitamin C Serum
1 Dark Colored Glass Dropper Bottle

½-1 tsp L-Ascorbic Acid Powder (I use "Solgar" brand)

1 tbsp Distilled Water

1 tsp Vegetable Glycerin (I use NOW brand)

1 drop Citrus Essential Oil Orange or Tangerine (optional)

Start by heating the water in the microwave for 20-30 seconds. Add L-ascorbic powder and mix vigorously until it dissolves (30 seconds). Then add the glycerin and continue to stir. Some of the crystals will still remain undissolved, so use a spoon or funnel to get your mixture into your bottle. Add your drop of oil after the serum mixture is in the bottle, and shake.

Use: The crystals will reappear and separate over time, so you must always shake before use. The hot water does slightly decrease the strength of the vitamin C, but it also absorbs better this way. Apply 5-10 drops to cleansed and toned skin. You will feel some mild tingling or stinging when you first apply it, since it is a raw form of the powder (especially if you exfoliate prior). This should subside after 30 seconds or so. You may also experience some mild redness initially—this is increased circulation. If you experience extreme redness or burning, rinse your face and discontinue use.

Since this is a low cost recipe (total supplies: $20) you can make many batches and use this on your body, too, since it also has had damage and needs repair and protection. One part L-ascorbic powder, 4 parts water, 1 part glycerin. Make small batches and use your DIY Vitamin C Serum quickly.

Multivitamin: Make the serum "multivitamin" by adding the contents of a vitamin E capsule and/or vitamin A capsule to the glycerin before mixing it with the aqueous water and vitamin C solution.

LYS Facial Cleansing Oil

1 ounce Castor Oil

1 ounce Carrier Oils

5-10 drops Essential Oil(s)

Combine oils in a bottle and shake. This is the ratio for normal and sensitive skin types. Oily and acneic skin: use 1 ½ ounces castor oil and ½ ounce carrier oil(s). Premature aging and dry / mature skin: use ½ ounce castor and 1 ½ ounce carrier oil(s). Castor oil can be drying. It is very thick. Oils will separate.

Use: Apply a quarter sized amount to the palm of your hand. Spread in hands and apply to DRY skin. This is your FIRST cleanse, so apply right on top of makeup, and massage lightly. Next, get a very warm, damp wash cloth and apply to face to remove oil and makeup. Rinse and repeat until face is clean. You may follow up with your regular cleanser for your SECOND cleanse. Use eye makeup remover if necessary. (Refer to the Love Lesson "Au Naturel" for the carrier and essential oils to use for your skin type.) I also use this oil in the shower as a facial moisturizing oil. If you don't like the castor oil, try combining equal parts Soy, Sesame, and Peanut oils, plus your essential oils, as an alternative.

LYS Hydrating Toner (All Skin Types)
2 ounces or ¼ cup Distilled Water

1 ounce or ⅛ cup Witch Hazel or Aloe Vera Juice

1 tbsp Aloe Vera Gel

1 tsp Vegetable Glycerin

6 drops Essential Oil (optional)

Combine all ingredients in a plastic bottle or spray bottle and shake well. You can vary this recipe as it is quite foolproof. Add a pinch of sea salt if you have acneic skin (keep away from eyes and lips). Mist face or apply with cotton pad. I like this homemade recipe better than my traditional toners.

LYS Almond Honey Facial Scrub (Non-Reactive Skin Only)
⅛ cup Ground Almonds

⅛ cup Ground Oatmeal

1 tbsp Whole Wheat Flour

1 tbsp Honey

2 tbsp Aloe Vera Gel or Vegetable Glycerin

1 tsp Kaolin (Clay) Powder (oily and acneic skin)

217

Mix ingredients together. I recommend only using this in the shower, as it is very messy. Your skin will be very smooth. Avoid contact with eyes and hair line.

LYS Pumpkin Enzyme Facial Exfoliant (All Skin Types)
½ cup Cooked or Canned Pumpkin Puree

½ tsp Cinnamon

2 tbsp Honey, Glycerin, or Aloe Vera Gel

Mix ingredients together and apply to skin. Let sit 8 minutes for sensitive skin (eliminate cinnamon), and up to 15 minutes for oily and acneic skin. Pumpkin contains natural enzymes which exfoliate, brighten, and reduce fine lines and wrinkles. For non-reactive skin, make it a scrub by adding ½ cup Sugar. Dry / mature skin: add 1 tsp of any Carrier Oil.

LYS Facial Masque for Dry and Sensitive Skin
1 Ripe Banana

½ Ripe Avocado

2 tbsp Honey

Mix ingredients and apply to face and neck. Allow to sit for 15 minutes, then rinse with lukewarm water. Add ½ tsp of any Carrier Oil for drier skin types. Add 2 tbsp whole or ground Oatmeal for sensitive or irritated skin. Add 2 tbsp Cocoa Powder for prematurely aging skin.

In Love With My Body Scrub
1 cup White or Brown Sugar

¼ cup Vegetable or Carrier Oil

15 drops Essential Oil(s)

1 tbsp Coconut Oil (optional)

1 tbsp Honey (optional)

Mix ingredients together (I like to use a chopstick to stir my recipes). Consistency should be like frosting: not too thick, not too thin. You can use any type of vegetable oil—see the carrier oils in the previous Love Lesson. I have even used Smart Balance brand cooking oil. It is a canola, soy, and olive blend. Add of your choice of essential oils. Grapefruit oil is cheerful for summer months, plus it helps with cellulite. Peppermint is festive during the holidays, and soothes sore muscles. This scrub makes a great gift. You can even keep a jar of it next to the sink as a hand scrub. Usage: The scrub must be done on dry skin to be effective. Stand on a dry towel (in the shower) and scrub your entire body from your neck down to your toes. Don't skip any area. Scrub until your skin flushes with circulation. Then shower. Be sure to keep the towel on the shower floor, or you may slip. This is my favorite recipe! Your skin will feel like velvet. Do this at night before you slip into bed with your significant other…so they can love your skin, too!

Like a Glove Body Oil
2 ounces Castor Oil

2 ounces Olive or Almond Oil

20 drops of your favorite Essential Oil

Combine ingredients and shake. This is a very heavy oil but it does the trick. Apply at the end of your shower to your entire body. Towel dry, and the oil will absorb into your skin, but remain soft throughout the day. Be sure to avoid getting it in your hair!

Goodbye Cellulite Oil
1 ounce Carrier Oil like Safflower, Olive, or Almond

15 drops of one or a blend of Essential Oils: Rosemary, Cypress, Juniper, Geranium, Juniper, Fennel

Shake oil before use. Rub vigorously into affected areas daily.

Natural Tooth Whitener
1 tbsp Baking Soda

1 tbsp Fresh Lemon Juice

or

1 tsp Toothpaste

1 tsp Baking Soda

1 tsp Hydrogen Peroxide

½ tsp Water

I know these are not a skin care recipes, but your teeth are on your face! I use both recipes, as I have very sensitive teeth and cannot use the store bought or professional tooth whiteners.

Use: Recipe 1: Mix baking soda and lemon juice together in a small bowl (This is intended for one use, only). Dip your toothbrush into the mixture, which will be very runny, and then brush your teeth. Just don't expect it to taste very good! It will get a little messy, so you may want to place a wash cloth or paper towel under your lower lip.

Continue dipping your brush, and applying for 2-3 minutes. Then rinse your mouth with water. I love the results, and it only needs to be done once a month. Yes, the lemon is acidic, but once a month should not damage your teeth, unlike store bought or professional whiteners that are done daily. You can use a store-bought fluoride rinse to seal the teeth's enamel.

Use: Recipe 2: Mix all ingredients together and brush for 2-3 minutes. I use this one in the shower!

LYS Lip Scrub
1 tsp Honey

1 tsp Sugar (Cane or Brown)

A pinch of Cinnamon

Mix together in a small container or bowl. Rub vigorously onto clean, dry lips and rinse. Your pout will be super soft and plump! It's safe to eat, too! (This can also double as a facial scrub for non-reactive skin types. Use in the shower after cleansing.)

Don't forget to refrigerate, label (and date) your Do-It-Yourself skin care products. They look like food, someone may mistake them for something to eat!

Love Lesson #29

Feed Your Skin

"Does what we eat affect our skin?" This is a question people have been asking for a long time. The simple answer is, "Yes." Yes, because the skin derives its nourishment from the blood stream, and the blood stream carries nutrients from the foods we eat and supplements we take. Your blood carries water, oxygen, food and secretions to your cells which are necessary for proper function. It also carries waste away from your skin cells.

Without question, what we eat affects our skin. The more nutrients in your blood stream, the healthier your skin will be. I am not a nutritionist, but as an aesthetician I must understand how to properly feed the skin. Instead of giving you a "diet" you must add to the list of others regimens you are trying to follow, I will instead list the top foods that contain essential nutrients for healthy skin (And my favorite recipe to get them: Love Your Skin "LYS" smoothie!).

SKIN LOVING NUTRIENTS

Silicon

An essential trace mineral for skin, hair, and nails. Important in the formation of connective tissues (collagen and elastin). Improves skin problems. Silicon deficiencies can result in wrinkles and sagging skin. 5-10mg per day.

Brown rice, Rice bran, Rolled Oats, Soybeans, Alfalfa, Bell Peppers, Beets, Leafy Greens, Pumpkins, Carrots, Onions, Cabbage, Cucumber, Cherries, Apples, Oranges, Raisins, Fish, Honey, Nuts and Seeds, Hard Water.

Vitamin A

Vital in the roles of maintenance, repair, and protection of skin cells. Prevents acne. RDA (recommended daily allowance) is 5000IU.

Meat: Liver.

Fruits and Vegetables: Sweet Potatoes, Carrots, Kale, Turnip Greens, Mustard Greens, Dandelion Greens, Collard Greens, Spinach, Butternut Squash, Red and Green Leaf Lettuce, Dried Apricots, Cantaloupe.

Dried Herbs and Spices: Parsley, Oregano, Basil, Marjoram, Paprika, Cayenne Pepper, Chili Powder.

Vitamin B Complex

Essential for healthy skin and healing. RDA is 1.4-30+ mg depending on the B vitamin.

Nuts: Pine, Pistachio, Macadamia, Pecans, Almonds, Peanuts, Hazelnuts, Filberts.

Plants: Edamame (Soy Beans), Rice and Wheat Bran, Sun-Dried Tomatoes, Sesame Butter, Sunflower Seeds,

Most Dried Herbs & Spices, Mushrooms, Avocados, Garlic, Asparagus, Pinto and Garbanzo Beans (Chickpeas), Bean Sprouts.

Meats: Liver, Pork Chops, Chicken, Bacon, Beef, Lamb.

Fish: Mackerel, Fresh Atlantic Salmon, Trout, Tuna, Anchovies, Swordfish, Caviar, Cod, Crab, Lobster.

Dairy: Eggs, Whey Powder, Cheese.

Misc: Yeast Extract, Molasses.

Vitamin C

Common co-factor in the production of collagen, and a powerful reducer of reactive oxides (free radicals). Inhibits irritants (potentially cancer causing) from entering cells.

RDA is 90mg-2000mg per day.

Red and Green Chili Peppers, Guava, Parsley, Kiwi, Broccoli, Brussels Sprouts, Papaya, Strawberries, Oranges, Kale, Lemon, Melon, Cauliflower, Limes, Garlic, Cabbage, Spinach, Mandarin Oranges, (Many other fruits and vegetables contain lesser amounts.)

Vitamin D

Required for proper cell growth and immune functions. RDA is 6,000IU, but is thought to be more like 10,000-40,000IU.

Cod Liver Oil, Sushi (raw fish specifically), Canned Fish, Oysters, Caviar, Tofu and Soy Milk, Ham, Salami, Sausage, Fortified Dairy, Eggs, and Mushrooms.

Vitamin E

Protects cells from elements that produce cell damaging free radicals. Regulates vitamin A in the body. RDA is 20mg.

Sunflower Seeds, Almonds, Pine Nuts, Peanuts, Dried Oregano and Basil, Paprika, Red Chili Powder, Dried Apricots, Green Olives, Cooked Spinach, and Cooked Tarot Root.

Vitamin K

Protects against Cancer, RDA is 80 micrograms, however there is no known toxicity, so you can fill up on it!

Fresh and Dried Herbs: Basil, Sage, Thyme, Parsley, Marjoram, Oregano, Coriander, Chili Powder, Curry, Paprika, Cayenne.

Fruit and Vegetables: Kale, Collard Greens, Spinach, Lettuce, Swiss Chard, Green Onions, Brussels Sprouts, Broccoli. Asparagus, Cabbage, Pickles, Prunes.

Zinc

Protects against skin lesions. RDA is 15mg.

Meat and Seafood: Oysters, Veal, Liver, Roast Beef, Lamb, Crab.

Plant: Dark Chocolate, Wheat Germ, Cocoa Powder, Peanuts; Pumpkin, Squash and Watermelon Seeds.

Copper

Required for connective tissue production. RDA is 2mg.

Meat and Seafood: Liver Pate, Oysters, Calamari, Lobster.

Plant: Sesame and Tahini Butter, Cocoa Powder and Chocolate, most Nuts, Sunflower Seeds, Sun Dried Tomatoes; Roasted Squash and Pumpkin Seeds

Dried Herbs: Basil (highest), Oregano, Marjoram, Savory, Parsley.

Calcium

Protects against skin cancer, promotes cellular health, encourages healthy skin pigmentation. RDA is 1000mg (best obtained from food sources rather than in supplement form).

Dried Herbs: Savory, Celery Seed, Dill, Marjoram, Rosemary, Sage, Parsley, Spearmint, Poppy Seed.

Plant: Sesame Seeds, Tofu, Almonds, Flax Seeds, Brazil Nuts.

Dairy: Low-fat Yogurt and Milk, Cheese: Parmesan, Romano, Gruyere, Mozzarella, Swiss, Cheddar, Goat Cheese, Provolone.

Fish: Herring

Omega 3's

Anti-inflammatory and can regulate hormones. They can alleviate dry, itchy skin.

Fatty Fish, Fish Oil, Flaxseeds, Flaxseed Oil, Walnuts, Pumpkin Seeds, Beans, and Avocados.

Lecithin

Protects cellular membranes and increases metabolism. Moisturizes and hydrates skin, internally. RDA for men 500 mg, women 425 mg. Can be taken in supplement form.

Fish, Egg Yolks, Soybeans, Cabbage, and Cauliflower.

Choline (B Vitamin)

Helps regulate water, fat, nutrients, and waste coming in and out of cells.

Plant: Soybeans, Peanuts, Potatoes, Lentils, Cauliflower, Oats, Sesame and Flax Seeds, Spinach, Swiss Chard, Collard Greens.

Meat and Dairy: Egg Yolks, Butter, Grain-fed Beef, Chicken, Shrimp, Turkey.

More Skin Loving Foods

Brown Rice: rich in Selenium, lifts mood, and fights breakouts.

Coffee: in moderation, contains antioxidants and elevates mood and brain function.

White Tea and Pomegranate: contain antioxidants.

Kale, Brussels sprouts, Cabbage, Cauliflower, Bok Choy, Broccoli and other leafy greens are "cruciferous" vegetables that contain phytochemicals with anticancer properties.

Dieting

As I have stated before, I believe in balance. I believe in living life on your terms. For this reason, I recommend the Weight Watchers program because it allows you to eat as many fruits and vegetables as you like—they're free! Many other diets restrict your fruits and veggies, and I don't like that. The Weight Watchers system supports whole grains, low fat and high protein, whether you are vegan, vegetarian, or a meat eater. It rewards you for exercise and is more of a health management program than a diet. It allows for wiggle room. I use Weight Watchers (online) to maintain my weight and healthy eating habits and have no other affiliation with their company. If you are looking for a more specific diet for skin only, I've included some in the Resources section at the end. It all boils down to eating clean and nutritiously, and restricting processed foods, preservatives and additives. Always take a multivitamin and mineral supplement.

Skin Loving Supplements

Youth Builder® Dietary Supplement $49.50 www.Murad.com

Naturally Clear Oral Supplement www.Drugstore.com or www.Amazon.com

My favorite way to get my skin loving nutrients is with a smoothie! There are endless combinations you can make, and they're quick, easy, and fun. I use a "Ninja" brand blender, I swear by it, as it blends better than a traditional blender since food doesn't get trapped in the blades. It is worth the investment, and they have models anywhere from $40-$200 at department stores and online. Here are several of my favorite recipes and their variations:

LYS Fruit Enzyme Smoothie
Boosts cell production and protection.

Base: 1 cup fresh Pineapple

1 ripe Banana

2-4 fresh Kale Leaves

6-10 ounces natural unfiltered Apple Juice

1 cup Ice

Chop and combine ingredients in your blender. You can substitute the juice with water, or ½ juice, ½ water to lessen the sugar.

Optional Additions: Strawberries, Blueberries, Raspberries, Blackberries, Kiwi, Mango, Carrots (shredded or baby), or any other sweet fruit or veggie to vary the flavor. You can also give it a boost by adding 1 tsp of Coconut oil—it adds to the sweet, tropical flavor.

Substitutions: Spinach, Swiss Chard, or any other green leafy vegetable, but Kale is the highest in vitamin C. This smoothie is only 2-4 Weight Watcher points depending on the amount of Apple Juice you use.

LYS Super Protein Power Smoothie
Supports building blocks of cells.

Base: 1 cup unsweetened Greek Yogurt or Soy Yogurt

1 ripe Banana

⅛ cup whole grain Oats (uncooked)

5-7 Raw Almonds

2 cups Ice

Zero calorie natural Sweetener (Truvia, Ideal, Nectresse, Stevia, et cetera) or Honey to taste

Flavor it by adding either: ½ tsp Cinnamon or Nutmeg, 1 tbsp Cocoa Powder, or 1-2 tbsp Peanut or other Nut Butter.

Combine ingredients, blend, and enjoy! This smoothie is 6-8 Weight Watchers points depending on the additions.

Love Lesson #30

Friends With

Benefits

There comes a point when you can only do so much yourself, and you need some extra TLC from a friend! The same can be said of your skin. When you feel like your at-home routine just isn't enough, it's time to find some friends with benefits for your skin. There are three types of individuals that can give your skin what it needs: aestheticians, nurses, and physicians (including dermatologists and plastic surgeons). How do you know who to see and when?

The differences are these: Dermatologists and physicians treat diseases and conditions of the skin; plastic surgeons offer procedures to change and improve the look of your features and skin; nurses can administer injections, and regenerative skin treatments like peels, microdermabrasion, and laser treatments; aestheticians do not treat conditions or inject, but rather treat skin care concerns and perform treatments to improve skin's health and appearance. The regulations on some treatments such as microdermabrasion and laser procedures vary by State. I believe you should layer the levels of Friends with Benefits in this order:

1. You: at-home regimen

2. Aesthetician treatments

3. Nurse

4. Physician or Dermatologist

5. Plastic Surgeon

It is not advisable to do nothing for your skin and then go to a plastic surgeon and expect them to fix what's wrong. You just won't have optimum results. Make sure you are using all the steps and services from the friends listed above in a chronological sequence. This will ensure your skin gets what it needs from all its friends.

Aesthetician / Spa Treatments

Aestheticians perform facial treatments on the skin, while dermatologists perform medical procedures. Quite often, women see a dermatologist when what their skin needs could likely be handled by an aesthetician. LYS Rule of Thumb: Visit an aesthetician before you see a dermatologist. Many women are still unfamiliar with the value of the services aestheticians can provide.

Facials, unless you've had a real one, usually conjure up images of a woman sitting in a chair having products slapped on her face, like you may have seen at the department store. If you've had a facial before, you know they are not only a relaxing slice of heaven, but also very effective in changing your skin.

The very first facial I had changed my mind completely about the power of skin care. I was in my mid twenties, and I had small bumps and breakouts covering my entire forehead. I wasn't having much success with what I was using at home or with the prescription medication from my doctor. The aesthetician at the spa where I worked (as a massage therapist at the time) talked me into having a facial. I thought I had been transported to another place in time, as she systematically applied products and steam towels to my skin. She used a rotary brush, and gently extracted the debris from my pores with her tools and tissue covered fingers. When the facial was finished, I was absolutely floored; the bumps were gone from my forehead! In one hour's time—my skin was magically transformed. Yes, the power of a professional facial is vastly underestimated.

Your aesthetician will customize the facial treatment to meet your skin's exact needs. They have an entire arsenal of products and facials tailored for every skin care issue. They also offer chemical peels and non-surgical facial rejuvenation procedures like LED photo facials, and microcurrent skin tightening and lifting. I recommend aestheticians as the first Friend with Benefits you call upon. Then move on to a medical spa or dermatologist if they cannot meet your skin's needs.

Aestheticians' services are the most affordable, ranging from $35-$120 per treatment. Find one that specializes in skin concerns, specifically. Not all aestheticians are created the same, and some just provide cookie cutter facials at resorts or day spas, without getting to know your skin on a one-on-one basis. Ask around for recommendations.

Aestheticians can also help you establish your at-home skin care regimen. This will take out the guess work for you, and they will be someone you can go to with any questions you have. Aestheticians are trained to refer to a dermatologist when they see anything of concern.

Many aestheticians offer a free skin care consultation, with no strings attached. Call several spas in your area and set up an appointment at each one. Once you develop a good relationship with your aesthetician, they can recommend how often you need a facial or a rejuvenation treatment. The rule of thumb is to book a facial with the change of seasons, or every 3-4 months. Four facials a year…you deserve it, and so does your skin.

Nurse / Medical Spa

Med spas and skin rejuvenation centers generally provide services that require the supervision of a nurse or physician, but are still cosmetic in nature, meaning they do not treat diseases and disorders of the skin—but they provide services like Botox ™ and filler injections, and all types of laser treatments for pigmentation, broken capillaries, and extreme premature aging. They also offer microdermabrasion, Thermage®, and even mini-facelifts.

The services at a med spa or skin rejuvenation center usually come with a higher price tag and range from $200-$2500, depending on the service. The services are usually sold in packages and require multiple sessions over a period of weeks or months.

Love Note: You may not be required to buy a package of visits, and can request paying for the individual sessions as you go, if you want to see how your skin will respond to treatment. This is how I have tried the different lasers and regenerating treatments at these centers.

Intense Pulsed Light (IPL) lasers are very effective in treating couperose skin—skin with excessive broken capillaries and redness. The laser uses heat to coagulate the superficial blood vessels, which are broken and not needed there. Another setting of the same laser is drawn to the areas of excessive pigment in the skin and stops the overproduction of the pigmented cells. Both conditions, however, can return if you continue to expose your skin to the damaging elements, and you must use the proper skin care regimen like antioxidants and SPF to strengthen and repair your skin so the conditions do not return.

Fillers and injections can treat deep lines that are not diminishing with skin care, alone. However, the fillers do fade over time, and can be over-filled, and then you have to wait them out. Some fillers now include ingredients that aim to stimulate collagen and elastin production in the area, which is what you want to be doing to your entire face with all the anti-aging recommendations. This will lift and re-build your skin's tissues, which will lessen lines. The last thing you want is thin skin with puffy fillers.

You will want to seek out a professional at a med spa after you are already using a proper at-home regimen, and have seen an aesthetician. Do not abuse your skin or fail to care for it, and go to a med spa for a quick fix. If you do this, the problems you are having will return and your dis-satisfaction will persist.

Dermatologist

Your skin will benefit from a physician friend when you have a condition that needs medicine or a medical proce-dure such as psoriasis, dermatitis, moles, skin lesions, cystic acne (deep within the skin), rashes, allergies, or anything causing concern that is non-cosmetic. Dermatologists treat diseases, and obviously have many years of education and experience to do so. Dermatologists are in the business of medicine, not skin care. Do not confuse the two. In cases of non-cystic acne, anti-aging, and skin rejuvenation, your best bet is to have them treated in a non-medical setting.

If you want your skin to function better, you have to take care of it. It could be compared to never brushing your teeth at home and only going to a dentist when you end up with a cavity or worse. I am not anti-dermatologist, or try-ing to be the Skin Care Nazi. I am pro skin care education, so that women are better equipped to make decisions that will give them healthy skin and keep them out of the doctor's office. I keep drilling this concept, because too often I meet clients who have not yet embraced this mentality, and are continually frustrated with their skin.

For example, I had a client and her teenage daughter who saw me for waxing services. The daughter had chronic breakouts, excessive oiliness, and irritated skin. For as long as I had been their aesthetician (over four years), the daughter had been seeing a dermatologist who had her on antibiotics and a topical, retinoid based acne medication. I could see that the daughter's pores were clogged and in need of extractions. I also knew that the drugstore brand products she was instructed to use by the dermatologist were not doing anything for her skin. However, her mother would never allow me to give the daughter a facial or recommend our professional grade products, citing that she must "ask the dermatologist first." The answer from the derm was always, "NO." Unfortunately, the daughter continued to have breakouts. I wonder how many young women are suffering from acne, when a facial every few months and the recommendations of an aesthetician could remedy the situation. The same holds true for other concerns like anti-aging and skin sensitivities. The best results can be obtained when aesthetician and physician are working together.

Plastic Surgeon

I heard the best advice from a plastic surgeon when asking him when a woman should "have work done." His advice was to "wait as long as possible, since you should only have one facelift in your lifetime (if you do, at all) and to wait until you have done absolutely everything else you can for your skin, it is as healthy as you can get it, and surgery is your last resort."

Remember, plastic surgery and procedures that "nip and tuck," lift, implant, and remove do not improve or repair the function of your skin, they only change the appearance of it. If you care for your skin through proper nutrition and regimen, you may never need surgery. If you only rely on surgery to fix the issues, we all know where that leads... Reality TV has blessed us with plenty of examples.

Love Note: Every day, at home, you have two opportunities to change your skin: morning and night. Don't waste them! The products you put on your face twice a day (if you are using good ones), accumulated, can make more of a difference than a quick trip to a Friend With Benefits. It will ensure that your skin is in the healthiest condition it can be. Then, when necessary, see a professional. Their treatments will work much better if you are already caring for your skin properly.

When you are in need of a Friend with Benefits, make sure you pick the right friend. They all have different skills you can appreciate, however they will all claim their services and treatments to be the best. It is hoped that this information helps you to make the right choice for your skin, not ones based on preconceived notions of who can care for it. When in doubt, keep a large circle of Friends with Benefits, and have an aesthetician, nurse, and physician friend on hand.

Love Lesson #31

Expert Tips

Here are some additional savvy tips the pros know, that will save you time, money, and help you Love Your Skin:

Custom Blend Your Products

You can enhance the properties and effectiveness of any of your skin care products by adding to them. We've already touched on this throughout the book, but I recommend doing it on a regular basis. Here's how:

Products you can add to:

Cleansers

Toners

Exfoliants

Moisturizers

Masques

SPF

Makeup

Body Lotion

Body Wash

Shampoo and Conditioner

Ingredients to add:

1-3 drops or pumps of your Serum.

1-5 drops Essential oils per ounce of product.

Carrier oils: 5-10 drops per ounce for heavier oils, and 1 tsp for lighter weight oils, per ounce of product.

Vitamins A, E, and C: Buy vitamin A and E oil capsules and L-ascorbic powder at your local health food store and add contents of capsule or 1/8 tsp powdered C, per ounce of products, for an antioxidant boost.

Liquid Mineral Makeup to your moisturizer or SPF.

Several drops of Water to your moisturizer.

Sea Water is very healing to troubled skin, full of minerals, and has antiseptic properties. Make your own sea water by adding a ¼ teaspoon sea salt, to 1 tablespoon hot water and stir until dissolved. Add the solution to your toner, or add a few drops to your moisturizer, when applying. This doesn't contain all the minerals found in seawater, but can be beneficial to acneic and problem skin.

You can add the new ingredients right into the container, or you can save your old makeup and skin care containers, then custom blend in them for each use. Don't be afraid to experiment. It's like making a cocktail for your skin!

Tapping

No, not tap dancing! "Tapotement" is the technical term for what I am calling "Tapping," and is a method used by pros in two different ways: to ward off Botox™ by relaxing the muscles, and to drive products into your skin.

Tap Your Botox™ Muscle: Do you have frown lines between your brows? All Botox™ does is "paralyze" the muscle so you can't use it. Often lines and wrinkles form in areas where the muscles are being used a lot. It's like lifting weights—the more you do it, the bigger and stronger the muscle gets. If you stop working out, the muscle gets smaller, right? So if you can become conscious of when you are frowning, stop doing it, and "tap" on the area with your fingers—the muscle will relax, and the lines that formed around it will diminish.

You may think this sounds crazy, and perhaps you would just rather get the Botox™, but tapping does work, if you do it. I became aware of this idea when I was 27, and started "tapping" the area between my brows daily, whenever I felt myself tensing it. I tap the number of my age. Ten years later, I do not need Botox™.

If you already use Botox™, and keep making the frowning expression, your scowl lines will return when the Botox™ wears off. Tap with your middle finger, with a decent amount of pressure. You can also tap with all of your fingers around your eyes to lessen crow's feet. Tap your forehead to relax the horizontal lines there. Tap the nasal labial lines along either side of your mouth, and around the entire mouth, to lessen the expression lines here. Do it when you are watching TV, making dinner, getting ready to fall asleep...whenever! I was doing it once, in my car at a stop light, and I looked over at a family in the car next to me, who all had very bewildered expressions on their faces. I only tap in private now!

Tap like you are playing the piano by alternating your fingers, or tap with all of them at the same time. Train yourself to keep your forehead and eyebrows relaxed. Scowling and frowning are not attractive expressions to make, anyway. A relaxed face is a beautiful face.

Tap Products Into Your Skin: It helps to drive them further down, and it firms and tones your face. Tap your serums and moisturizers after you've applied them. Tap for about 30 seconds all over your face with the piano technique or with all fingers, paying special attention to the trouble spots. Have fun with it!

Facial Exercises

Since we are on the topic of facial muscles... What happens to your body if you don't exercise it? It loses its muscle tone and shape, right? The same things happen to your face. I do not expect you to use any funky gadgets—just do these five facial movements that will engage, stretch, and tone your facial muscles and also enhance blood flow. They are actually yoga stretches for the face. Do them anytime, but at least once a day. They only take 15 seconds to do!

Make each movement, then hold for 3 seconds.

1. Pout Face: Scrunch up all the muscles of your face towards the center, like an angry pouting child. Hold.

2. Left Stretch: Move the left side of your mouth (face), over towards your right ear, until you feel the muscles in your face stretch. Hold.

3. Right Stretch: Move the right side of your mouth (face), over towards your left ear, until you feel the muscles in your face stretch. Hold.

4. "O": Open your mouth like you are making a big "O" shape with your mouth, until you feel your facial muscles moving downward. Hold.

5. The Caveman "E": Make an "E" movement with your mouth, carefully jutting your lower jaw forward until you feel the muscles of your lower jaw, chin, and neck, stretch. Hold. This is a muscle we no longer use, that the cavemen used to tear meat from the bone. It needs to be exercised and will tone your double chin, or prevent you from getting one!

6. The Gene Simmons (Bonus): Stick your tongue all the way out like KISS. Open your mouth wide, then stick out your tongue. (Some people may feel silly doing this, so I added it as a bonus!)

Massage Your Face On a Daily Basis

Massage firms the underlying tissues and tones muscles! Who doesn't want that? Massage increases blood flow to your skin which brings in nutrients, oxygen, and carries away toxins. It removes excess fluids which cause puffiness and sagging. Facial muscles need massage because the face receives less blood flow and exercise than the other areas of our body.

There are two types of massage I am recommending. They only take a few minutes a day and will drastically lift and tone your face. One is done daily in the shower. The other is done several times a week, when you are lying down. (If you have cystic acne, very sensitive skin, or broken capillaries, avoid the shower massage, and only do the acupressure massage until your skin is healthier (and it will be).

All massage movements should be done in an upward, outward, or inward motion—never downward. You want to move against gravity, or against the direction that the lines form, to counteract them.

Here's an easy way to incorporate massage into your daily Skin Ritual, and it only takes 30 seconds! This massage starts at your neck and works its way up the face towards the hairline.

Facial Shower Massage

1. Apply cleanser (creates slip).

2. Make your hands into fists. Use the flat surface of your knuckles and fingers (the part you would use to punch someone with) to do the massaging. Move slowly, but press firmly, through the tissues towards the bone, to reach the muscles.

3. Neck: Start at your neck and move your fists up towards your jawbone. 2x.

4. Jaw: Start at the middle of chin and run both fists outward, along jaw line towards ears. 3x.

5. Cheeks: Start at jawbone (next to ears) and move fists upward, over cheeks, to eyes, moving through the contours of your cheeks. 2x.

6. Repeat above, just on inner face, next to both sides of lips.

7. Start at corners of mouth and move outward towards ears (horizontally). 2x.

8. Repeat above step, now from next to your nose, outward towards your ears. 2x.

9. Eyes: Use the pad of your ring finger (or a knuckle) and circle your eye area. Make a clockwise circle around your right eye, and a counterclockwise circle around your left. 3x.

10. Forehead: Roll one or both fists from eyebrows, upward towards your hairline. 3x.

11. Massage your temples. 10 circles.

You're finished! This will literally take 30 seconds to do. (I timed it.) It will take years off your face, keep your skin healthy, lifted, and toned—if you do it daily, or 3x a week minimum.

The next massage can be performed on all skin types. It helps release tension that causes blockages in circulation and healthy functions. It releases pressure in the sinuses and helps relieve headaches. This massage starts at the forehead and works its way down the face, towards the jaw bone. It is done on dry skin (unless you want to add a drop or two of essential oils to your hands). You will be using the pads (tips) of your thumbs and ring fingers, mainly. You want to use heavy pressure.

Acupressure Massage

1. Forehead: Place your thumbs next to each other between your eyebrows. Press down, firmly (towards the bone), and hold for 2 counts. Now, move up one space towards your hairline, and press again. Continue upward to hairline. 2x.

2. Start between both brows with both thumbs again, this time pressing a horizontal line outward, towards temples. Move in upward rows to cover entire forehead.

249

3. Upper Eyes: Use your thumbs on the upper eyes. Press first under brow bone, at inner corner of eye, and move outward as you go (like you are digging your thumbs into your eye socket). Press and hold each spot for 2 counts.

4. Under Eyes: Now do same as above, only working from outer corner of eye, inward towards nose. Press into the bone of your eye socket. Use ring finger.

5. Temples: Press and hold for 6 counts.

6. Cheek Bones: Press with thumbs, under cheek bones, from next to corner of nose, and follow cheek bone outward towards ear. Press thumbs in and up. Repeat.

7. Lips: Press into the depression above your upper lip. Press down into your teeth, using your thumb. Press into the space underneath your lower lip on your chin.

8. Jaw: Place your thumbs together at the tip of chin. Move outward along the jaw line towards ears. Press and hold for 2 counts. Repeat. Next, press and hold the muscle of your jaw (by ears) for 6 seconds.

You are finished! You can do this anytime. Just make sure both your hands and face are clean. It only takes a few minutes. Your face will thank you.

Product Hide and Seek

Don't hide your products away! This may seem like a common sense statement, but I believe it is the missing link in many women's skin care routine. It's the old "Out of sight, out of mind" thing. If you have a "product shelf" or "product drawer," you will know what I'm talking about. You buy a product, or many products, with the best intentions to use them…and you forget to, because they're hidden away.

I suggest—no, insist—that you devote an area in your bathroom for your products exclusively. I know many of us have limited space in the bathroom. Don't let this stop you. Go out and buy a wall shelf, cabinet, or table that you can fit in there, somehow. Or consider a cute decorative basket on the bathroom counter, to hold all the products you are currently using; this way you won't be able to ignore them! Remember, they can't work if they are in a drawer or a shelf. They can only work if they're on your face!

Love Lesson #32

Stressed Out

Think of your skin as an expression of what's within. Whatever is happening on the inside will show up on the outside. Whether it's toxins, disease, hormonal and glandular imbalances, malnutrition, dehydration, or stress, it will be reflected in your skin. Please pay attention to it. The blood that travels through your organs and bodily systems is what nourishes your skin and tells it everything that's going on internally.

Your overall health and nutrition are extremely important. It's easy to understand the role a disease, disorder, or other health concern plays in our well being, but one thing we often overlook and let run rampant in our lives is stress.

We know how stress makes us feel mentally and emotionally, but the effects of stress are devastating to our physical being and play a huge role in the health of our skin. The easiest example I can give you is what I call "Wedding Skin." It can happen to both brides- and grooms-to-be, but mainly to women. I have treated many brides' skin before their nuptials over the years, and have seen this issue countless times. The stress of planning a wedding can last for months, if not years, and this chronic tension causes our body to release hormones and secretions in an attempt to help us cope. These secretions spike many of our glands' activity like sweat and oil (when referring to the skin). As mentioned in the Love Lesson on acneic skin, spikes in testosterone, androgen, and estrogen can directly and indirectly increase Sebaceous (oil) gland activity. The stress also causes our body to produce the destructive free radicals we dislike. The shock of stress on our central nervous system lowers our body's immune system's ability to fight off the aggressors. All of these things, when mixed together, can show up on your skin as cystic acne, dermatitis (irritation), rashes, pimples, infection and more. When you are stressed, your body sends blood to your heart, lungs, and brain, and vital organs, resulting in less blood flow to your skin, leaving it sallow and without the necessary oxygen and nourishment we've been discussing.

I had a client who was simultaneously going through a divorce, attending school full-time, working full-time, and raising two teenagers on her own. It all made its way to her face: she had extreme redness, itching, regular acne, cystic acne, and peeling, all on her face, neck, chest, and back. The stress she was under was so overwhelming that it caused her to become allergic to herself—or more specifically, the stress. Her body was producing a histamine (allergic) response to the stress.

In the cases of "Wedding Skin" or "allergies" to stress, the only thing that will stop the skin problems and other issues it's causing is to get rid of the stress. I know that may sound too simple, or easier-said-than-done, but if the stress is too much for your skin to handle, there's a good chance it's more than you should be handling, too.

If you can't get through, or out of, the situation imme-diately, it's essential to find ways to help you contend with it. Just recognizing what the stress is doing to you is the first step, and creating ways to keep the stress out is the next. Do whatever helps you release the tension and anxiety. Have a good laugh, cry, or yell; dance, sing, breathe, go for a run or walk, take a hot bath, cook, clean, write, have a glass of wine, shop, see a doctor or therapist, work out, do whatever you can do.

Stop, take some deep breaths, and don't let the stress into your body and mind. There is always next time to ap-proach a new situation, knowing the effects stress can have on you, and to keep it out. Then the evidence of internal health, happiness, and wellbeing will be the glow that shows through in your skin.

A Lifetime of Love… I know many women view their skin care routine as a chore…one extra thing they must do to end their day or get it started. In addition to everything else on your "To Do" list, taking care of your face can eas-ily get skipped.

My hope is that this book has empowered you with in-formation and tips which will make the time you spend with your face a more pleasurable and rewarding experience. Time that is positive and productive, when you know that what you are doing is the proper care for your skin. This knowledge will help you have a healthy relationship with your skin and love it for all the years to come....

Congratulations!

You can now say…

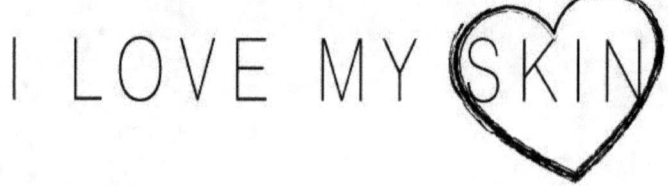

Thank you for reading Love Your Skin: Expert Secrets Exposed!

If you enjoyed Love Your Skin, please recommend it to a friend and share your review on Amazon.com and GoodReads.com, so other readers can love their skin, too. Thank you!

If you have any concerns or issues with the eBook formatting of this book, please email: info@mogulpress.com

Do you have a question or skin care secret of your own you'd like to share? Nicci Leigh would love to hear from you!

Email: loveyourskin@niccileigh.com

Website: www.NicciLeigh.com for Contact Information, Social Media links, Mailing List, Updates, Videos, and more.

Many similar recipes, recommendations and products can also be found on Nicci Leigh's **"Love Your Skin" Pinterest board:**
http://pinterest.com/princessbitch/love-your-skin-expert-skin-care-secrets-exposed-co/

Other Books By Nicci Leigh:

<u>Princess B*tch: The Sassy Guide to Relationships, Power, and Success</u>

TIRED OF EVERYONE ELSE RULING YOUR WORLD? IT'S TIME TO TAKE IT BACK! Reclaim your feminine power and use it in ways you never thought possible — this sassy, easy-to-use guide for all women will help you to be happy, successful, and satisfied. It will change the way you look at your relationships, your career, it will connect you to your feminine power and change your life. "Princess Bitch" is a fun, easy-to-read, guide for all women. The world NEEDS powerful women. When you complete all 13 Princess Bitch Golden Rules you will be UNSTOPPABLE!

Money Bags: A Breast Implant Experience. One Woman's Intimate Journey.

In this petite memoir, best-selling women's author Nicci Leigh shares her lighthearted yet deeply personal struggle with self-esteem, relationships, and body image, highlighting questions and concerns many women face today.

Nicci bares all in this intimate narrative in hopes of reaching other women who may be experiencing similar issues, or would just like to read about a topic that could use a little light shed on its rather taboo stigma: that of our bodies (breasts), and how they affect the way we feel about ourselves.

It's honest, witty, and totally forthcoming!

VISIT WWW.NICCILEIGH.COM FOR LINKS TO ALL VENDORS.

References

Books:

Gerson, Joel. D'Angelo, Janet. Lotz, Shelley. *Milady's Standard Fundamentals for Estheticians, Ninth Edition.* New York, Delmar Learning. 2004

Winter, Ruth M.S. *A Consumer's Dictionary of Cosmetic Ingredients, Fifth Edition.* New York, Three Rivers Press. 1999

Lee, William H. D.S.C, R. Ph. and Lee, Lynn CN. *The Book of Practical Aromatherapy.* Keats Publishing Inc. 1992

Elizabeth, Stephanie. *The Real Guide to Flawless Skin: Only 4 Weeks to Clear Skin.* Stephanie Elizabeth. 2010-2012

Websites:

www.wikipedia.com

www.FDA.org

www.thebeautybean.com

www.sassybella.com

www.organicconsumers.org

www.fitsugar.com

www.TLC.com

www.mightynest.com

www.shesknows.com

www.cosmeticinfo.org

www.thenaturalhaven.com

www.care2care.com

www.skinacea.com

www.lexli.com

http://iverson.cm.utexas.edu

www.breastcancerfund.org

www.realself.com

www.whfoods.com

www.yourdailyfix.com

www.ehow.com

Resources

Nutrition:

The Clear Skin Diet by Alan C. Logan

Eating for Beauty by David Wolfe

The Water Secret: The Cellular Breakthrough to Look and Feel 10 Years Younger by Howard Murad

Anti-Aging By Choice: Smoothies to Look and Feel Younger by Sandra Douglas

Eating Clean in a Dirty World: An Easy to Follow Guide to Cleaning up Your Diet for Life by Jennafer Ashley

www.weightwatchers.com

Do-It-Yourself Skin Care:

The Complete Idiots Guide to Making Natural Beauty Products by Sally W. Trew, Zonella B. Gould

Organic Body Care: 175 Homemade Recipes for Glowing Skin and Vibrant Self by Stephanie Tourles

www.essentialwholesale.com Bulk Cosmetic Ingredients

www.ewg.org/skindeep/ Product Ingredient Database

Fitness and Wellness:

The Sivananda Guide to Yoga: A Complete Guide to the Physical Postures, Breathing Exercises, Diet, Relaxation,

and Meditation Techniques of Yoga by Sivananda Yoga Center and Vishnu Devananda
The 60 Second System: Burn Fat Lose Weight Build Muscle in Just 60 Seconds by Sharon Moore

Style and Self (to go with your new skin!):
The Little Black Book of Style by Nina Garcia
Princess Bitch: The Sassy Guide to Relationships, Power, and Success by Nicci Leigh www.NicciLeigh.com
What Smart Women Know by Steven Carter and Julia Sokol

Essential Oils:
The Complete Book of Essential Oils and Aromatherapy by Valerie Ann Worwood
www.YoungLiving.com

Naturopathic Physician available for online consultations:
www.drnoel.fixyournutrition.com

Miscellaneous:
www.cosdna.com Product and Ingredient Database

Index

My Love Affair

With Skin Care

It was love at first sight. The first memory I have of true infatuation and desire was of a cosmetic product. Makeup, actually. Tiny tubes and shiny plastic cases of vibrantly colored creams, sticks, and powders were organized by type in a tackle or craft box, of sorts, on my grandmothers' vanities. At age four, this makeup was more than mere face paint to me: it was the only thing I wanted.

Both my grandmothers owned these cosmetic tackle boxes, and both boxes were completely off limits to me, except for the several times I was allowed to touch the bright coral cream rouge and electric blue eye shadow, under their close supervision. I dreamt of those boxes, I conceived of ways to get near them—alone with them, all to myself. I had to, of course, settle for the generic nail polish and makeup kits made for children, which never had enough pigment, and dissatisfied me completely. I begged and pleaded with the Grandmas until I at least got to sit and stare at the boxes.

This should give you some idea of the beginning to my abnormal obsession with beauty products. I already knew then, at that tender age, that cosmetics would always be one of the few things closest to my heart.

Several years later, my "little girl world" got a lot bigger when we moved from my family's apartment to a new house in a suburban neighborhood. Cosmetics would soon play a much larger role in my life than I could have imagined. That big house, in that big neighborhood, must have become a magnifying glass on my parents' already troubled marriage, and they soon separated. My mother was left broken hearted, trying her best to raise a daughter and make a house payment on her own—so she hired Mrs. Engle. She was a middle aged woman from the neighborhood who would babysit me—essentially raise me—while my mother worked as a personal banker. Mrs. Engle was (of course) an Avon Lady. Her home, which consisted of herself, her husband, and their two adult children, was the quintessential "normal" that my home was lacking. So, I spent most of my time there. Correction: all of my time, in her spare bedroom which housed her Avon product inventory.

I pored over every cleanser, cream, tube, spray; you name it, I knew every ingredient, shade or scent that it came in. I memorized the catalogs and organized the samples. At seven years old, my innocence was stripped by a broken home, but my passion was in full effect (and became my therapy).

Mrs. Engle and I decided that I would become the neighborhood's Avon Lady, and assume all duties under her account and name. While the other girls in the neighborhood were at ballet class or playing with their dolls, I was traipsing door to door with catalogs, orders, and samples in tow. All the neighbor women embraced me and welcomed me as their "new" Avon consultant. I effortlessly recited the latest products and seasonal offers, and at times, received more orders than Mrs. Engle and I could keep up with. I soon heard that several of the other moms "disapproved" of the new girl with the divorcing parents and Avon route. I didn't mind. I found the cosmetics much more intriguing than ballet and dolls.

I don't recall the end of my Avon career, but I do remember that at age ten my mother and I left the big house in the suburbs for a small house on an acre in the country, and two years later, puberty arrived. My ill-fated genetic predisposition to my mother's oily and acneic skin was soon realized. Keep in mind, during my entire cosmetic obsession I was never allowed to wear makeup, and I was not a "girly" type at all. In my spare time I was quite a tomboy—I rode a dirt bike, and was content to own several pairs of jeans and a few shirts. The "cosmetic thing" (I've assumed) was my destiny.

Throughout my teens, skin care became the polar opposite of the magical escape it had been during my childhood. It became an endless search for anything that would clear the chronic breakouts I was experiencing. Nothing worked. I would often accept invitations to sleep over at a friend's house, not for "girl time," but for the opportunity to secretly rummage through their mother's beauty drawer or shelf in search of something I hadn't yet tried. On rare oc-

XV

casions a scrub, emulsion, or lotion did the trick and my skin would clear for a day or two, only, to return to the pimples and blotches soon after.

I can recall many trips on the weekends to the local mall's cosmetic counters, where my mother would discuss products for what seemed like hours with the woman in the white lab coat, while I peered into the backlit glass shelves of cosmetic heaven. She was also on the eternal hunt for a cream or potion to control her own oil prone, acneic skin.

This battle my mother and I both fought, I know, was not unique to us alone, but it was one we never won. My teenage acneic years extended into my twenties, and my lifetime as a young woman was colored by my hatred for cosmetics that did not work. Not for me, anyway.

Fast forward to two children and a divorce later, and I now was my mother, working full time to support my family, and still battling my skin. I was fed up. I was done trying dermatologists, medications, and home remedies. I knew I needed an education, and my skin's destiny was in my hands, alone. In 1999 the state of Michigan licensed the cosmetology division of Esthetics, and by 2003 I was enrolled in a program. I excelled immediately, and had visions of myself as a skin care extraordinaire, with my own spa, and clients coming to me for my skin care omniscience.

Fast forward once again to a degree in Esthetics, a teaching degree in skin care, a private practice since 2003, a trainer for over five of the top professional product lines, a college level educator, a spa owner with a private skin care line, to becoming an author.

Did you catch everything in that last part? I tried to spare you the details there, but essentially my love and acclimation for cosmetics from that young age grew into an understanding of how to treat my clients' and my own skin care concerns. I never had perfect skin. I would never have learned how to treat others' if I hadn't needed to fix my own. Skin, which I now love, by the way!

Nicci

Acknowledgements

I would like to extend my appreciation to:

My Beta readers: Brooke Martin, Janice Duff, Geri Mazza, Azziza Salem, Ashlee Yuile, Kristina Balish, and Kathy Smith, for your support. Thank you for your time.

To Marcus Bieth for your friendship and design talents. To Justin H. Phillips for your editing skills. I am still slaughtering the comma…

To deLancey Moser at REN skincare, Mary Koster with Rodan & Fields, Jeanine Maroudis, Tracey Burke with Kiehls, Courtney at Aveda, and the staff at L'Occitane Somerset North for your time and generosity.

To Fedra West at Phaedra Elise Photography for the best shutter skills! Thank you April Headley for your creative contribution. Nevaeh Livingston for your assistant skills.

To my family, friends, and clients who showed their support: you always have a place in my heart. To my husband, Aaron Smith, for your patience and common sense insight through each book I write.